CALIFORNIA STATE UNIVERSITY, SACI

Th

Clinics in Developmental Medicine No. 140

FEEDING THE DISABLED CHILD

© 1996 Mac Keith Press
526/529 High Holborn House, 52–54 High Holborn, London WC1V 6RL

Senior Editor: Martin C.O. Bax
Editor: Pamela A. Davies
Managing Editor: Michael Pountney
Sub Editor: Pat Chappelle

Set in Times and Avant Garde on QuarkXPress

First published in this edition 1996

British Library Cataloguing-in-Publication data:
A catalogue record for this book is available from the British Library

ISSN: 0069 4835
ISBN: 1 898683 08 5

Printed by The Lavenham Press Ltd, Water Street, Lavenham, Suffolk
Mac Keith Press is supported by **Scope** (formerly The Spastics Society)

Clinics in Developmental Medicine No. 140

Feeding the Disabled Child

Edited by

PETER B. SULLIVAN
John Radcliffe Hospital
Oxford

LEWIS ROSENBLOOM
Alder Hey Children's Hospital
Liverpool

with a Foreword by
JAMES F. BOSMA
University of Maryland School of Medicine
Baltimore, MA

1996
Mac Keith Press

Distributed by 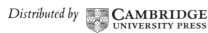 CAMBRIDGE
UNIVERSITY PRESS

CONTRIBUTORS

Janet H. Allaire, MA

Assistant Professor of Pediatrics, University of Virginia School of Medicine, Kluge Children's Rehabilitation Center, Charlottesville, VA, USA

Peter A. Blasco, MD

Associate Professor of Pediatrics, University of Minnesota School of Medicine, Minneapolis, MN, USA

Lesley Carroll, MRCSLT

Specialist Speech and Language Therapist, Cheyne Child Development Service, London, England

Graham Clayden, MD, FRCS

Reader in Paediatrics, United Medical and Dental School of Guy's and St Thomas' Hospital, London, England

Robin P. Glass, MS, OTR

Occupational Therapist, Children's Hospital and Medical Center, *and* Clinical Assistant Professor, Department of Rehabilitation Medicine, University of Washington, Seattle, WA, USA

David A. Lloyd, MChir, FRCS

Professor of Paediatric Surgery, University of Liverpool *and* Alder Hey Children's Hospital, Liverpool, England

Eric Loveday, MB, BS, MRCP, FRCR

Consultant Radiologist, Southmead Hospital, Bristol; *and* Honorary Senior Lecturer, University of Bristol, England

Agostino Pierro, MD, FRCS

Senior Lecturer in Paediatric Surgery, University of London; *and* Consultant Paediatric Surgeon, Great Ormond Street Hospital for Children, London, England

Sheena Reilly, BAppSc, PhD

Specialist Speech and Language Therapist, Great Ormond Street Hospital for Children, London, England

Lewis Rosenbloom, FRCP — Consultant Paediatric Neurologist, Alder Hey Children's Hospital, Liverpool, England

Ben (N.J.) Shaw, MD, FRCP — Consultant in Neonatal and Respiratory Medicine, Liverpool Women's Hospital, Fazakerley Maternity Hospital and Alder Hey Children's Hospital; *and* Honorary Lecturer, University of Liverpool, England

Virginia A. Stallings, MD — Chief, Nutrition Section, Children's Hospital of Philadelphia; *and* Associate Professor, University of Pennsylvania School of Medicine, Philadelphia, PA, USA

Richard D. Stevenson, MD — Associate Professor of Pediatrics, University of Virginia School of Medicine, Kluge Children's Rehabilitation Center, Charlottesville, VA, USA

Peter B. Sullivan, MA, MD, MRCP — University Lecturer and Honorary Consultant Paediatrician, University of Oxford, Department of Paediatrics, John Radcliffe Hospital, Headington, Oxford, England

Lynn S. Wolf, MOT, OTR — Occupational Therapist, Children's Hospital and Medical Center, *and* Clinical Assistant Professor, Department of Rehabilitation Medicine, University of Washington, Seattle, WA, USA

Babette S. Zemel, PhD — Director, Nutrition and Growth Laboratory, Children's Hospital of Philadelphia; *and* Clinical Assistant Professor of Pediatrics, University of Pennsylvania School of Medicine, Philadelphia, PA, USA

CONTENTS

CONTRIBUTORS   *page* *v*

FOREWORD   *ix*
James F. Bosma

1. INTRODUCTION: AN OVERVIEW OF THE FEEDING DIFFICULTIES
   EXPERIENCED BY DISABLED CHILDREN   1
   Peter B. Sullivan and Lewis Rosenbloom

2. THE DEVELOPMENT OF EATING SKILLS IN INFANTS AND YOUNG
   CHILDREN   11
   Richard D. Stevenson and Janet H. Allaire

3. THE CAUSES OF FEEDING DIFFICULTIES IN DISABLED CHILDREN   23
   Peter B. Sullivan and Lewis Rosenbloom

4. THE NUTRITIONAL AND NEURODEVELOPMENTAL CONSEQUENCES
   OF FEEDING DIFFICULTIES IN DISABLED CHILDREN   33
   Lewis Rosenbloom and Peter B. Sullivan

5. THE RESPIRATORY CONSEQUENCES OF NEUROLOGICAL DEFICIT   40
   Ben (N.J.) Shaw

6. THE THERAPEUTIC APPROACH TO THE CHILD WITH FEEDING
   DIFFICULTY: I. ASSESSMENT   47
   Lynn S. Wolf and Robin P. Glass

7. NUTRITIONAL ASSESSMENT OF THE DISABLED CHILD   62
   Virginia A. Stallings and Babette S. Zemel

8. DIAGNOSTIC IMAGING AND SPECIAL INVESTIGATIONS IN THE
   ASSESSMENT OF THE DISABLED CHILD   77
   Eric Loveday

9. DROOLING   92
   Peter A. Blasco

10. CONSTIPATION IN DISABLED CHILDREN   106
    Graham Clayden

11. THE THERAPEUTIC APPROACH TO THE CHILD WITH FEEDING
DIFFICULTY: II. MANAGEMENT AND TREATMENT   117
Lesley Carroll and Sheena Reilly

12. THE THERAPEUTIC APPROACH TO THE CHILD WITH FEEDING
DIFFICULTY: III. ENTERAL FEEDING   132
David A. Lloyd and Agostino Pierro

13. THE ETHICS AND IMPLICATIONS OF TREATMENT PROGRAMMES
FOR DISABLED CHILDREN WITH FEEDING DIFFICULTIES   151
Lewis Rosenbloom and Peter B. Sullivan

INDEX   157

FOREWORD

This monograph records important advances in the understanding and care of feeding and nutrition problems in neurologically impaired children. Earlier, such feeding problems, and related malnutrition and growth failure, were accepted as ordinary concomitants of these children's disorders. In recent years, however, dysphagic children have profited from increasing clinical attention. There has been a convergence of clinicians in various disciplines: physicians, dentists, speech and occupational therapists, nutritionists, psychologists and others, and in some places they are joined as teams in the evaluation and management of children impaired in feeding and in nutrition.

Clearly, the contributors to this volume are writing from extensive experience. They are aware of the complexity of the ingestion performance, that its oral, pharyngeal and esophageal stages interact though they differ in physiology and, thus, in mechanisms of impairment. The impairments, primary in one or more stages, may secondarily affect the competence of another stage.

The oral stage of feeding is distinctive in the role of sensation and perception in its actions. Sensory impairments may be at the root of oral disorders such as excessive accumulation of oral content and labial spill (drooling), as well as distortion of food delivery into the pharynx.

The writers recognize that the upper alimentary tract, of the pharynx and esophagus, is a two-way street; gastroesophageal reflux and esophagopharyngeal regurgitation are latent liabilities in various patterns of feeding disorder.

The processes of ingestion and respiration intersect at the pharynx. If food enters the pharynx without elicitation of swallow, or if swallow incompletely empties the pharynx or leaks food into the larynx, or if esophageal or gastric content is returned to the pharynx, the child is liable to acute or chronic lower respiratory disease.

The necessity of adequate nutrition is a theme recurrent in various chapters. Chronic malnutrition impairs neurologic and general somatic development and compounds the motor impairment of feeding and of other actions. Maintenance and repair of nutrition may require direct enteral feeding, although gastrostomy feeding may occasion other problems of reflux and of dumping. The decision about oral versus direct enteral feeding may be difficult for the clinician, the parents and the child; these interactions are thoughtfully considered in the book.

We who work with dysphagic children are grateful, on behalf of these children, for an up-to-date collection of information, understanding and wisdom about their feeding and nutrition. We particularly appreciate the unravelling of primary and secondary elements in this complex matter of feeding. We are grateful, too, that adequate attention has been given to the secondary elements, such as the pleasures and satisfactions of eating, and to the adverse complications such as drooling, constipation, lower respiratory diseases and malnutrition. In many dysphagic children and families, these derivative elements are of greater concern than the difficulties in eating. Because of this collection, these children and their families can be better understood as persons interacting with defined disabilities, and treatment and day-to-day management can be approached with defined goals.

JAMES F. BOSMA, MD
Research Professor
Department of Pediatrics
University of Maryland School of Medicine
Baltimore, MA, USA

1
INTRODUCTION: AN OVERVIEW OF THE FEEDING DIFFICULTIES EXPERIENCED BY DISABLED CHILDREN

Peter B. Sullivan and Lewis Rosenbloom

Breathing and eating are two of the most fundamental and vital of human activities. The anatomical structures which subserve the functions of sucking, chewing, swallowing and respiration are in close physical proximity, provide a conduit for both food and air, and require complex and highly integrated levels of neuromuscular control. Coordination of sucking, chewing, swallowing and breathing is essential to the prevention of aspiration of food and swallowing of air, and to the efficient intake of nutrients.

Disability and feeding
The development of oral-motor skills mirrors general neurological maturation. In order to attain optimum oral-motor skill a child must have the ability to move oral and facial structures independently of the rest of the body (Ottenbacher *et al.* 1983*a*). Control of the axial skeleton is also important, as proper body position is essential to promote normal feeding (Mueller 1975, Morris 1989). Furthermore, in order to become competent feeders, children must be able to use their arms and hands adroitly, with coordinated hand-to-mouth movements, and be sufficiently dextrous to use forks, spoons or chopsticks as extensions of their own hands. Not surprisingly, insults to the developing brain can have dramatically deleterious effects on a child's ability to feed. Lack of independent mobility and inability to ask for food or express preferences further contribute to the difficulties that disabled children have in obtaining an adequate intake of nutrients. In addition, behavioural problems are common in disabled children, and meal times may become a focus for the expression of these, thus further compromising feeding (Palmer *et al.* 1975, Riordan *et al.* 1984, Ottenbacher *et al.* 1985).

Social consequences of feeding difficulties
We eat not simply for the purpose of maintenance and growth of our bodies but also as a fundamental social activity shared with others. Failure of an infant to suck properly may be the mother's first indication that there is something wrong with her child (Weiss 1988, Reilly and Skuse 1992). The disabled child may become for the parents, as Goldie (1966) put it, the living grave of their hoped-for normal baby, and the family's capability of adapting to this disappointment will be reflected in the quality of the mother–child relationship and particularly in the feeding relationship (Weir 1979, Sloper and Turner 1993). Adaptation to a child with disability is an ongoing process throughout the child's life rather than an

event accomplished in the first months after diagnosis (Sloper and Turner 1993). Some parents may lack the necessary personal skills to achieve this adaptation.

Early in their development children spend a great deal of time exploring the environment with their mouths. This exploration serves a dual purpose: firstly, to gather information from the outside world, and secondly, to desensitize the mouth to different textures and tastes (Ottenbacher *et al.* 1983*a*). Children with abnormal tone and abnormal facial sensitivity respond to the touch of food and feeding utensils with increased muscle tone and abnormal oral patterns. These abnormal reactions make food intake extremely difficult and increase the risk of choking and vomiting. Meal times with disabled children can be prolonged and stressful, with both caretakers and children becoming frustrated and anxious (Johnson and Deitz 1985, Reilly and Skuse 1992). Children with severe oral-motor dysfunction can take from six to 18 times longer to eat a mouthful of food than normal children (Gisel and Patrick 1988, Ohwaki and Zingarelli 1988, Croft 1992). On average, mothers of disabled children spend 3½ hours per day feeding their child as compared to 0.8 hours for mothers with normal children; some mothers spend over 7½ hours a day trying to feed their disabled child (Johnson and Deitz 1985). Even long meal-times do not compensate for the severity of these children's feeding impairment and they frequently become malnourished.

Feeding disabled children, therefore, can be unrewarding and unenjoyable, especially with children who have a tendency to vomit over themselves and their caretaker (Morris 1989). Mothers may be unable to leave their disabled child in anyone else's care for fear that they will be unable to cope at meal-times. The difficulties with feeding such a child impose severe restrictions on the activities and opportunities for the mother both within and outside the home (Hirose and Ueda 1990). The situation is further complicated by negative feelings generated by the child's obvious failure to thrive and inability to reward the mother by returning affection. Thus, mothers tend to assume the major responsibility for feeding the disabled child (Hirose and Ueda 1990), while fathers often take a more passive role and may feel less confident with the child and also resentful of the restriction on joint activities between husband and wife. Reilly and Skuse (1992) using a videotape study noted the lack of verbal interaction and very mechanical manner in which disabled children were often fed by their mothers. The enormous burden of feeding their children as perceived by the mothers is reflected by the high levels of probable psychiatric disturbance suggested by several reports (Weir 1979, Breslau *et al.* 1982, Hirose and Ueda 1990, Reilly and Skuse 1992, Sloper and Turner 1993).

Nutrition
The prevalence of growth disorders and nutritional deficits in disabled children is unknown. What data there are available suggest that around a third (13–52 per cent) of such children are significantly undernourished (Hammond *et al.* 1966, Roberts and Clayton 1969, Wallace 1972, Palmer *et al.* 1975, Thommessen *et al.* 1991). In the majority of these studies growth retardation was most closely associated with inadequate intake as a result of self-feeding impairment and oral-motor dysfunction. The association between the severity of cerebral palsy (CP) and dysphagia and oral-motor impairment has been clearly demonstrated (Krick and Van Duyn 1984, American Dietetic Association 1992). Waterman *et al.* (1992)

2

studied 56 children with CP and found that 15 (27 per cent) had evidence of dysphagia and 44 (78 per cent) had a significant degree of drooling. More recent unpublished data suggests that the magnitude of this problem may be considerably greater. Questionnaires completed for the Family Fund in the UK indicate that 81 per cent of 11,794 children with CP experienced feeding difficulties of some degree (M. Bax 1995, personal communication).

The suboptimal nutrition resulting from inadequate intake is not without its consequences. In addition to linear growth failure there is a decrease in muscle strength (Russell *et al.* 1983), which in the respiratory system reduces the effectiveness of the cough reflex and predisposes to aspiration pneumonia (Efthimiou *et al.* 1988) and in the limbs causes an increased circulation time, resulting in the cold, mottled peripheries frequently seen in wasted CP children (Patrick *et al.* 1986). Undernutrition is associated with a decrease in cerebral function (Stoch *et al.* 1982, Grantham-McGregor *et al.* 1991) with possible exacerbation of the existing neurological impairment. Chronic undernutrition may be associated with increased irritability, and decreased motivation and energy available for activities such as play and rehabilitation (Stallings *et al.* 1993). Significant developmental progress has been shown to accompany improved nutritional status (Sanders *et al.* 1990). CP children have an abnormal increase in total body water and extracellular water in comparison to healthy children. Both improvement in nutrition and, where possible, increased physical activity have been shown to decrease this abnormality (Berg 1973). Disturbances in the immune system secondary to malnutrition predispose these patients to infection, particularly of the lungs and the urinary tract. Furthermore, healing of pressure sores is delayed in children with malnutrition. In view of such diverse complications, it is apparent that correction of malnutrition is central to the management of neurologically disabled children.

Marked progress in the clinical management of disabled children has emerged from advances in medical and engineering technology, especially with respect to ambulation, communication, education and orthopaedic care. The same degree of input, however, has been lacking when it comes to nutritional care (Stallings *et al.* 1993). Growth failure and undernutrition have often been accepted as inevitable and irremediable consequences of CP. This is unfortunate as it is now evident that undernutrition in those with CP is often correctable (Patrick *et al.* 1986, Sanders *et al.* 1990). Even simply increasing the caloric density of foods offered has been shown to be effective in producing weight gain in disabled children with feeding difficulties (Evers *et al.* 1991). Patrick *et al.* (1986) not only demonstrated that wasting could be corrected in children with CP but their data also suggested that nutritional improvement was associated with improvement in the children's spasticity and affect. Rempel *et al.* (1988) also demonstrated that it was possible to improve the nutritional status of children severely affected by CP but observed that this did not eliminate growth retardation. Similarly, Sanders *et al.* (1990) noted that the earlier adequate nutritional management of children with severe CP is initiated, the more readily the nutritional deficits will reverse. Such evidence points to the possibility of a 'sensitive' or 'critical' period with respect to establishing normal feeding ability (Illingworth and Lister 1964, Blackman and Nelson 1985, Geertsma *et al.* 1985). Certainly there is evidence that delay in instituting oral feedings in children fed exclusively by nasogastric tube leads to oro-aversive behaviour which inhibits development of normal feeding (Palmer *et al.* 1975,

Morris 1989). Moreover, habituation to the presence of a nasogastric tube may induce a reduction in the activation of the gag reflex. This would further increase the risk of aspiration.

One of the central problems pertaining to the nutritional management of disabled children with feeding problems has been the lack of information about their precise dietary requirements. Estimated Average Requirements (EARs) are not applicable to children who are short for age or whose physical activity is impaired by motor dysfunction. Abnormal movements such as athetosis are a complicating factor which could potentially increase energy requirements (Phelps 1951). Conversely, those immobile individuals with spasticity who are at risk of obesity may require a lower calorie intake (Fonkalsrud *et al.* 1985). Little work, however, has been done to fully investigate these theoretical considerations. On behalf of The Spastics Society, Eddy *et al.* (1965) conducted a pilot study of dietary intakes and energy expenditure using indirect calorimetry and showed that the total energy requirements and intakes of CP children were less than those of normal children of the same age. As a result of physical deformity and growth abnormality, reduced weight for height cannot be relied on in the usual way as an indicator of wasting. As a consequence of these factors there are no appropriate growth standards for children with neuromuscular disability.

Culley and Middleton (1969) attempted to express caloric requirements of 52 severely disabled CP children in terms of body size and motor status instead of age. Their findings were that ambulatory children without motor dysfunction required 14.7 calories per centimetre of height per day, ambulatory children with motor dysfunction required 13.9 kcal/cm/day, and those who were nonambulatory required 11.1 kcal/cm/day. These workers, however, relied on measurement of height to estimate caloric needs, but children with CP frequently have scoliosis and contractural deformity which renders accurate measurement of height impossible. Measurement of limb length instead of height allows documentation of linear growth failure or growth failure associated with CP and provides a reliable measure of change in growth with nutritional therapy (Spender *et al.* 1989).

Children with mild CP who can walk are usually below average height, but are not malnourished. Very dependent disabled children, however, are short, underweight for stature, with wasted muscles and reduced skinfold thickness (*Lancet* 1990). There is abundant evidence that nutritional factors have a role in the growth failure and mortality of children with CP (Roberts and Clayton 1969, Patrick *et al.* 1986, Shapiro *et al.* 1986, Sanders *et al.* 1990) and that the magnitude of the impact of nutritional status on linear growth is proportional to disease severity (Hammond *et al.* 1966; Pryor and Thelander 1967; Berg 1973; Spender *et al.* 1989; Bandini *et al.* 1991; Thommessen *et al.* 1991*a,b*; Stallings *et al.* 1993). Nevertheless, the adverse effects of malnutrition superimposed upon severe disability have not been fully assessed (Culley and Middleton 1969), and the determinants of linear growth of severely disabled CP children remain to be defined (Shapiro *et al.* 1986). Moreover, growth failure in this group of children is probably multifactorial and not simply a matter of inadequate nutrition. This is indicated by the failure of aggressive nutritional therapy to reverse growth retardation especially when instituted in older children even before they have lost growth potential following skeletal maturation (Rempel *et al.* 1988). Gastrostomy feeding, for instance, may lead to an increase in weight and in fat stores without a concomitant acceleration of linear growth (Rempel *et al.* 1988, Stallings *et al.* 1993). It is likely that there are as yet unidentified neurophysiological mechanisms associated with the damage to the developing brain which also contribute significantly to the growth retardation (Roberts and Clayton 1969).

Implications for care

Nutritional management is thus an important part of the comprehensive care and rehabilitation of disabled children and contributes not only to better growth but also to improvement in physiological and functional capacity. To this end, multidisciplinary team care of such children is required and should include input from, amongst others, nursing, paediatrics, neurology, gastroenterology, paediatric surgery, speech therapy, dietetics, physiotherapy and occupational therapy (Palmer et al. 1975; Kenny et al. 1989; Pesce et al. 1989; Wodarski 1990, 1992; Boyle 1991; Reilly and Skuse 1992; Couriel et al. 1993). Diagnostic imaging and radiology also has an increasing part to play in the assessment of disabled children. Ultrasound studies of oral-motor function (Tuchman 1989) together with videofluoroscopic study of the swallowing process (Morton et al. 1993) have increased our ability to assess the potential for oral feeding and determine the optimum route by which to provide nutrition.

In conjunction with the information provided by imaging, speech therapists can evaluate the level of oral-motor functioning and institute oral-motor therapy if appropriate (Ottenbacher et al. 1983a). It is important to note, however, that the evidence that oral-motor therapy can be effective in improving nutritional intake is very scant and that it is important not to rely solely on this modality of treatment (Morris 1989). Although oral-motor therapy has become fashionable in recent years, and may improve use of the mouth and phonatory systems in exploration and sound play, there is, in fact, little evidence that it is effective either in terms of increased weight gain or improved oral-motor function for eating (Ottenbacher et al. 1981, 1983b; Morris 1989). As Shapiro et al. (1986) point out, 'those attempting to improve the oral-motor function of children with cerebral palsy must also monitor their patients' growth to identify children requiring adjunctive methods of feeding.'

Input from a dietitian is invaluable in assessing nutritional needs and advising on appropriate feeds and adjunctive methods of feeding. Gastroenterologists assist this process and also advise on treatment of constipation and gastro-oesophageal reflux (GOR). Numerous reports have demonstrated the association between neurological disability and clinically significant GOR (Eddy et al. 1965, Cadman et al. 1978, Jolley et al. 1978, Sondheimer and Morris 1979, Wesley et al. 1981, Byrne et al. 1982, Corbally et al. 1985, Schärli 1985, Spitz and Kirtane 1985, Halpern et al. 1991, Spitz et al. 1993). In the largest of these studies, Sondheimer and Morris demonstrated that 15/136 (11 per cent) of institutionalized children with severe retardation and recurrent vomiting had GOR. Several reasons have been proposed for this, including hiatus hernia (Abrahams and Burkitt 1970), adoption of a prolonged supine position (Halpern et al. 1991), and increased intra-abdominal pressure secondary to spasticity or scoliosis (Schärli 1985). Central nervous system dysfunction is likely to be the prime cause and have an impact on upper gastrointestinal motility. Papaila et al. (1989) reported that 28 per cent of children with symptomatic GOR had marked delays in gastric emptying. A reduction in the lower oesophageal sphincter (LOS) pressure in association with brain damage has been demonstrated both in animals (Vane *et al.* 1982) and in children (Sondheimer and Morris 1979, Berezin *et al.* 1986). Such incompetence in the LOS may not only predispose to GOR but also to occurrence of recurrent respiratory disease (Cadman *et al.* 1978, Christie *et al.* 1978, Euler *et al.* 1979). Furthermore, interference with the LOS pressure following gastrostomy tube placement (Jolley *et al.* 1986) may account for the observation that clinically significant GOR can develop in up to two-thirds of children following gastrostomy tube placement (Mollitt *et al.* 1985, Berezin *et al.* 1986, Grunow *et al.* 1989). Mollitt *et al.* (1985) observed that, while a feeding gastrostomy can greatly facilitate the care of the neurologically disabled child, postoperative follow-up for development of GOR was essential. In those subjects requiring a surgical antireflux procedure, follow-up is necessary as these carry significant postoperative morbidity in between 20 and 59 per cent of patients with up to 20 per cent requiring re-operation for recurrence of symptoms (Wesley *et al.* 1981, Wilkinson *et al.* 1981, Byrne *et al.* 1982, Spitz and Kirtane 1985, Vane *et al.* 1985, Dedinsky *et al.* 1987, Turnage *et al.* 1989).

Nutritional rehabilitation of disabled children can thus be associated with increased mortality (Raventos *et al.* 1982) and morbidity secondary to GOR or aspiration. It may also entail increased work for caregivers and increased costs of care. It is therefore necessary to document the impact of such rehabilitation on growth and quality of life for both patient and caregiver (Stallings *et al.* 1993). After reduced mobility, poor feeding ability is the best single predictor of early death in profoundly disabled individuals with mental retardation (Eyman *et al.* 1990). The extent to which this is directly due to malnutrition is uncertain. Oral-motor dysfunction clearly predisposes to aspiration, a significant degree of which occurs in around one-third of CP children (Helfrich-Miller *et al.* 1986, Griggs *et al.* 1989). It is also noteworthy that this is probably underestimated clinically, as cough is a poor indicator of aspiration in this group of children (Linden and Siebens 1983, Splaingard *et al.* 1988). It is perhaps not surprising that pneumonia is the leading cause of death in profoundly retarded individuals, accounting for between 30 and 50 per cent of all deaths (Cleland *et al.* 1971, Chaney *et al.* 1979).

The issues summarized in this chapter are discussed in detail in the remainder of this volume. Published research evidence and clinical experience form the basis of the views expressed by the contributors.

REFERENCES

American Dietetic Association (1992) 'Position of the American Dietetic Association: nutrition in comprehensive program planning for persons with developmental disabilities.' *Journal of the American Dietetic Association*, **92**, 613–615.
Abrahams, P., Burkitt, B.F. (1970) 'Hiatus hernia and gastro-oesophageal reflux in children and adolescents with cerebral palsy.' *Australian Paediatric Journal*, **6**, 41–46.
Bandini, L.G., Schoeller, D.A., Fukagawa, N.K., Wykes, L.J., Dietz, W.H. (1991) 'Body composition and energy expenditure in adolescents with cerebral palsy or myelodysplasia.' *Pediatric Research*, **29**, 70–77.
Berezin, S., Schwarz, S.M., Halata, M.S., Newman, L.J. (1986) 'Gastroesophageal reflux secondary to gastrostomy tube placement.' *American Journal of Diseases of Children*, **140**, 699–701.
Berg, K. (1973) 'Nutrition of children with reduced physical activity due to cerebral palsy.' *Bibliotheca 'Nutritio et Dieta'*, No. 19, 12–20.
Blackman, J.A., Nelson, C.L.A. (1985) 'Reinstituting oral feedings in children fed by gastrostomy tube.' *Clinical Pediatrics*, **24**, 434–438.

Boyle, J.T. (1991) 'Nutritional management of the developmentally disabled child.' *Pediatric Surgery International*, **6**, 76–81.

Breslau, N., Staruch, K.S., Mortimer, E.A. (1982) 'Psychological distress in mothers of disabled children.' *American Journal of Diseases of Children*, **136**, 682–686.

Byrne, W.J., Euler, A.R., Ashcraft, E., Nash, D.G., Seibert, J.J., Golladay, E.S. (1982) 'Gastroesophageal reflux in the severely retarded who vomit: criteria for and results of surgical intervention in twenty-two patients.' *Surgery*, **91**, 95–98.

Cadman, D., Richards, J., Feldman, W. (1978) 'Gastro-esophageal reflux in severely retarded children.' *Developmental Medicine and Child Neurology*, **20**, 95–98.

Chaney, R.H., Eyman, R.K., Miller, C.R. (1979) 'Comparison of respiratory mortality in the profoundly mentally retarded and in the less retarded.' *Journal of Mental Deficiency Research*, **23**, 1–7.

Christie, D.L., O'Grady, L.R., Mack, D.V. (1978) 'Incompetent lower esophageal sphincter and gastro-esophageal reflux in recurrent acute pulmonary disease of infancy and childhood.' *Journal of Pediatrics*, **93**, 23–27.

Cleland, C.C., Powell, H.C., Talkington, L.W. (1971) 'Death of the profoundly retarded.' *Mental Retardation*, **9** (5), 36.

Corbally, M.T., Simpson, E., Guiney, E.J. (1985) 'Management of gastroesophageal reflux in mentally retarded children.' *Irish Medical Journal*, **78**, 317–319.

Couriel, J.M., Bisset, R., Miller, R., Thomas, A., Clarke, M. (1993) 'Assessment of feeding problems in neuro-developmental handicap: a team approach.' *Archives of Disease in Childhood*, **69**, 609–613.

Croft, R.D. (1992) 'What consistency of food is best for children with cerebral palsy who cannot chew?' *Archives of Disease in Childhood*, **67**, 269–271.

Culley, W.J., Middleton, T.O. (1969) 'Caloric requirements of mentally retarded children with and without motor dysfunction.' *Journal of Pediatrics*, **75**, 380–384.

Dedinsky, G.K., Vane, D.W., Black, C.T., Turner, M.K., West, K.W., Grosfeld, J.L. (1987) 'Complications and reoperation after Nissen fundoplication in childhood.' *American Journal of Surgery*, **153**, 177–183.

Eddy, T.P., Nicholson, A.L., Wheeler, E.F. (1965) 'Energy expenditures and dietary intakes in cerebral palsy.' *Developmental Medicine and Child Neurology*, **7**, 377–386.

Efthimiou, J., Fleming, J., Gomes, C.,Spiro, S.G. (1988) 'The effect of supplementary oral nutrition in poorly nourished patients with chronic obstructive pulmonary disease.' *American Review of Respiratory Disease*, **137**, 1075–1082.

Euler, A.R., Byrne, W.J., Ament, M.E., Fonkalsrud, E.W., Strobel, C.T., Siegel, S.C., Katz, R.M., Rachelefsky, G.S. (1979) 'Recurrent pulmonary disease in children: a complication of gastroesophageal reflux.' *Pediatrics*, **63**, 47–51.

Evers, S., Munoz, M.A., Vanderkooy, P., Jackson, S.,Lawton, M.S. (1991) 'Nutritional rehabilitation of developmentally disabled residents in a long-term-care facility.' *Journal of the American Dietetic Association*, **91**, 471–473.

Eyman, R.K., Grossman, H.J., Chaney, R.H., Call, T.L. (1990) 'The life expectancy of profoundly handicapped people with mental retardation.' *New England Journal of Medicine*, **323**, 584–589.

Fonkalsrud, E.W., Ament, M.E., Berquist, W. (1985) 'Surgical management of the gastroesophageal reflux syndrome in childhood.' *Surgery*, **97**, 42–48.

Geertsma, M.A., Hyams, J.S., Pelletier, J.M., Reiter, S. (1985) 'Feeding resistance after parenteral hyperalimentation.' *American Journal of Diseases of Children*, **139**, 255–256.

Gisel, E.G., Patrick, J. (1988) 'Identification of children with cerebral palsy unable to maintain a normal nutritional state.' *Lancet*, **1**, 283–286.

Goldie, L. (1966) 'The psychiatry of the handicapped family.' *Developmental Medicine and Child Neurology*, **8**, 456–462.

Grantham-McGregor, S.M., Powell, C.A., Walker, S.P., Himes, J.H. (1991) 'Nutritional supplementation, psychosocial stimulation, and mental development of stunted children: the Jamaican Study.' *Lancet*, **338**, 1–5.

Griggs, C.A., Jones, P.M., Lee, R.E. (1989) 'Videofluoroscopic investigation of feeding disorders of children with multiple handicap.' *Developmental Medicine and Child Neurology*, **31**, 303–308.

Grunow, J.E., al-Hafidh, A-S., Tunell, W.P. (1989) 'Gastroesophageal reflux following percutaneous endoscopic gastrostomy in children.' *Journal of Pediatric Surgery*, **24**, 42–45.

Halpern, L.M., Jolley, S.G., Johnson, D.G. (1991) 'Gastroesophageal reflux: a significant association with central nervous system disease in children.' *Journal of Pediatric Surgery*, **26**, 171–173.

7

Hammond, M.I., Lewis, M.N., Johnson, E.W. (1966) 'A nutritional study of cerebral palsied children.' *Journal of the American Dietetic Association*, **49**, 196–201.

Helfrich-Miller, K.R., Rector, K.L., Straka, J.A. (1986) 'Dysphagia: its treatment in the profoundly retarded patient with cerebral palsy.' *Archives of Physical Medicine and Rehabilitation*, **67**, 520–525.

Hirose, T., Ueda, R. (1990) 'Long-term follow-up study of cerebral palsy children and coping behaviour of parents.' *Journal of Advanced Nursing*, **15**, 762–770.

Illingworth, R.S., Lister, J. (1964) 'The critical or sensitive period, with special reference to certain feeding problems in infants and children.' *Journal of Pediatrics*, **65**, 839–848.

Johnson, C.B., Deitz, J.C. (1985) 'Time use of mothers with preschool children: a pilot study.' *American Journal of Occupational Therapy*, **39**, 578–583.

Jolley, S.G., Johnson, D.G., Herbst, J.J., Pena, A., Garnier, R. (1978) 'An assessment of gastroesophageal reflux in children by extended pH monitoring of the distal esophagus.' *Surgery*, **84**, 16–24.

—— Tunell, W.P., Hoelzer, D.J., Thomas, S., Smith, E.I. (1986) 'Lower esophageal pressure changes with tube gastrostomy: a causative factor of gastroesophageal reflux in children?' *Journal of Pediatric Surgery*, **21**, 624–627.

Kenny, D.J., Koheil, R.M., Greenberg, J., Reid, D., Milner, M., Moran, R., Judd, P.L. (1989) 'Development of a multidisciplinary feeding profile for children who are dependent feeders.' *Dysphagia*, **4**, 16–28.

Krick, J., Van Duyn, M.A.S. (1984) 'The relationship between oral-motor involvement and growth: a pilot study in a pediatric population with cerebral palsy.' *Journal of the American Dietetic Association*, **84**, 555–559.

Lancet (1990) 'Growth and nutrition in children with cerebral palsy.' *Lancet*, **335**, 1253–1254. *(Editorial.)*

Linden, P., Siebens, A.A. (1983) 'Dysphagia: predicting laryngeal penetration.' *Archives of Physical Medicine and Rehabilitation*, **64**, 281–284.

Mollitt, D.L., Golladay, E.S., Seibert, J.J. (1985) 'Symptomatic gastroesophageal reflux following gastrostomy in neurologically impaired patients.' *Pediatrics*, **75**, 1124–1126.

Morris, S.E. (1989) 'Development of oral-motor skills in the neurologically impaired child receiving non-oral feedings.' *Dysphagia*, **3**, 135–154.

Morton, R.E., Bonas, R., Fourie, B., Minford, J. (1993) 'Videofluoroscopy in the assessment of feeding disorders of children with neurological problems.' *Developmental Medicine and Child Neurology*, **35**, 388–395.

Mueller, H. (1975) 'Feeding.' *In:* Finnie, N.R. (Ed.) *Handling the Young Cerebral Palsied Child at Home.* New York: E.P.Dutton, pp. 113–132.

Ohwaki, S., Zingarelli, G. (1988) 'Feeding clients with severe multiple handicaps in a skilled nursing care facility.' *Mental Retardation*, **26**, 21–24.

Ottenbacher, K., Scoggins, A., Wayland, J. (1981) 'The effectiveness of a program of oral sensory motor therapy with the severely and profoundly developmentally disabled.' *Occupational Therapy Journal of Research*, **1**, 147–160.

—— Bundy, A., Short, M.A. (1983a) 'The development and treatment of oral-motor dysfunction: A review of clinical research.' *Physical and Occupational Therapy in Pediatrics*, **3**, 1–13.

—— Hicks, J., Roark, A., Swinea, J. (1983b) 'Oral sensorimotor therapy in the developmentally disabled: a multiple baseline study.' *American Journal of Occupational Therapy*, **37**, 541–547.

—— Dauck, B.S., Gevelinger, M., Grahn, V., Hassett, C. (1985) 'Reliability of the Behavioral Assessment Scale of Oral Functions in Feeding.' *American Journal of Occupational Therapy*, **39**, 436–440.

Palmer, S., Thompson, R.J., Linscheid, T.R. (1975) 'Applied behavior analysis in the treatment of childhood feeding problems.' *Developmental Medicine and Child Neurology*, **17**, 333–339.

Papaila, J.G., Wilmot, D., Grosfeld, J.L., Rescorla, F.J., West, K.W., Vane, D.W. (1989) 'Increased incidence of delayed gastric emptying in children with gastroesophageal reflux. A prospective evaluation.' *Archives of Surgery*, **124**, 933–936.

Patrick, J., Boland, M., Stoski, D., Murray, G.E. (1986) 'Rapid correction of wasting in children with cerebral palsy.' *Developmental Medicine and Child Neurology*, **28**, 734–739.

Pesce, K.A., Wodarski, L.A., Wang, M. (1989) 'Nutritional status of institutionalized children and adolescents with developmental disabilities.' *Research in Developmental Disabilities*, **10**, 33–52.

Phelps, W.M. (1951) 'Dietary requirements in cerebral palsy.' *Journal of the American Dietetic Association*, **27**, 869–870.

Pryor, H.B., Thelander, H.E. (1967) 'Growth deviations in handicapped children. An anthropometric study.' *Clinical Pediatrics*, **6**, 501–512.

8

Raventos, J.M., Kralemann, H., Gray, D.B. (1982) 'Mortality risks of mentally retarded and mentally ill patients after a feeding gastrostomy.' *American Journal of Mental Deficiency*, **86**, 439–444.

Reilly, S., Skuse, D. (1992) 'Characteristics and management of feeding problems of young children with cerebral palsy.' *Developmental Medicine and Child Neurology*, **34**, 379–388.

Rempel, G.R., Colwell, S.O., Nelson, R.P. (1988) 'Growth in children with cerebral palsy fed via gastrostomy.' *Pediatrics*, **82**, 857–862.

Riordan, M.M., Iwata, B.A., Finney, J.W., Wohl, M.K., Stanley, A.E. (1984) 'Behavioral assessment and treatment of chronic food refusal in handicapped children.' *Journal of Applied Behavior Analysis*, **17**, 327–341.

Roberts, G.E., Clayton, B.E. (1969) 'Some findings arising out of a survey of mentally retarded children. Part II: Physical growth and development.' *Developmental Medicine and Child Neurology*, **11**, 584–594.

Russell, D.McR., Leiter, L.A., Whitwell, J., Marliss, E.B., Jeejeebhoy, K.N. (1983) 'Skeletal muscle function during hypocaloric diets and fasting: a comparison with standard nutritional assessment parameters.' *American Journal of Clinical Nutrition*, **37**, 133–138.

Sanders, K.D., Cox, K., Cannon, R., Blanchard, D., Pitcher, J., Papathakis, P., Varella, L., Maughan, R. (1990) 'Growth response to enteral feeding by children with cerebral palsy.' *Journal of Parenteral and Enteral Nutrition*, **14**, 23–26.

Schärli, A.F. (1985) 'Gastroesophageal reflux and severe mental retardation.' *Progress in Pediatric Surgery*, **18**, 84–90.

Shapiro, B.K., Green, P., Krick, J., Allen, D., Capute, A.J. (1986) 'Growth of severely impaired children: neurological versus nutritional factors.' *Developmental Medicine and Child Neurology*, **28**, 729–733.

Sloper, P., Turner, S. (1993) 'Risk and resistance factors in the adaptation of parents of children with severe physical disability.' *Journal of Child Psychology and Psychiatry*, **34**, 167–188.

Sondheimer, J.M., Morris, B.A. (1979) 'Gastroesophageal reflux among severely retarded children.' *Journal of Pediatrics*, **94**, 710–714.

Spender, Q.W., Cronk, C.E., Charney, E.B., Stallings, V.A. (1989) 'Assessment of linear growth of children with cerebral palsy: use of alternative measures to height or length.' *Developmental Medicine and Child Neurology*, **31**, 206–214. [Published erratum appears in *DMCN*, **32**, 1032.]

Spitz, L., Kirtane, J. (1985) 'Results and complications of surgery for gastro-oesophageal reflux.' *Archives of Disease in Childhood*, **60**, 743–747.

—— Roth, K., Kiely, E.M., Brereton, R.J., Drake, D.P., Milla, P.J. (1993) 'Operation for gastro-oesophageal reflux associated with severe mental retardation.' *Archives of Disease in Childhood*, **68**, 347–351.

Splaingard, M.L., Hutchins, B., Sulton, L.D.,Chaudhuri, G. (1988) 'Aspiration in rehabilitation patients: video-fluoroscopy vs bedside clinical assessment.' *Archives of Physical Medicine and Rehabilitation*, **69**, 637–640.

Stallings, V.A., Charney, E.B., Davies, J.C., Cronk, C.E. (1993) 'Nutrition-related growth failure of children with quadriplegic cerebral palsy.' *Developmental Medicine and Child Neurology*, **35**, 126–138.

Stoch, M.B., Smythe, P.M., Moodie, A.D., Bradshaw, D. (1982) 'Psychosocial outcome and CT findings after gross undernourishment during infancy: a 20-year developmental study.' *Developmental Medicine and Child Neurology*, **24**, 419–436.

Thommessen, M., Heiberg, A., Kase, B.F., Larsen, S., Riis, G. (1991a) 'Feeding problems, height and weight in different groups of disabled children.' *Acta Paediatrica Scandinavica*, **80**, 527–533.

—— Kase, B.F., Riis, G.,Heiberg, A. (1991b) 'The impact of feeding problems on growth and energy intake in children with cerebral palsy.' *European Journal of Clinical Nutrition*, **45**, 479–487.

Tuchman, D.N. (1989) 'Cough, choke, sputter: the evaluation of the child with dysfunctional swallowing.' *Dysphagia*, **3**, 111–116.

Turnage, R.H., Oldham, K.T., Coran, A.G.,Blane, C.E. (1989) 'Late results of fundoplication for gastro-esophageal reflux in infants and children.' *Surgery*, **105**, 457–464.

Vane, D.W., Shiffler, M., Grosfeld, J.L., Hall, P., Angelides, A., Weber, T.R., Fitzgerald, J.F. (1982) 'Reduced lower esophageal sphincter (LES) pressure after acute and chronic brain injury.' *Journal of Pediatric Surgery*, **17**, 960–964.

Vane, D.W., Harmel, R.P., King, D.R.,Boles, E.T. (1985) The effectiveness of Nissen fundoplication in neurologically impaired children with gastroesophageal reflux.' *Surgery*, **98**, 662–667.

Wallace, H.M. (1972) 'Nutrition and handicapped children.' *Journal of the American Dietetic Association*, **61**, 127–133.

Waterman, E.T., Koltai, P.J., Downey, J.C., Cacace, A.T. (1992) 'Swallowing disorders in a population of children with cerebral palsy.' *International Journal of Pediatric Otorhinolaryngology*, **24**, 63–71.

Weir, K. (1979) 'Psychological factors in feeding disorders occurring in mentally or multiply handicapped children.' *Child: Care, Health, and Development*, **5**, 285–294.

Weiss, M.H. (1988) 'Dysphagia in infants and children.' *Otolaryngologic Clinics of North America*, **21**, 727–735.

Wesley, J.R., Coran, A.G., Sarahan, T.M., Klein, M.D., White, S.J. (1981) 'The need for evaluation of gastro-esophageal reflux in brain-damaged children referred for feeding gastrostomy.' *Journal of Pediatric Surgery*, **16**, 866–871.

Wilkinson, J.D., Dudgeon, D.L., Sondheimer, J.M. (1981) 'A comparison of medical and surgical treatment of gastroesophageal reflux in severely retarded children.' *Journal of Pediatrics*, **99**, 202–205.

Wodarski, L.A. (1990) 'An interdisciplinary nutrition assessment and intervention protocol for children with disabilities.' *Journal of the American Dietetic Association*, **90**, 1563–1568.

2
THE DEVELOPMENT OF EATING SKILLS IN INFANTS AND YOUNG CHILDREN

Richard D. Stevenson and Janet H. Allaire

In normal infants and young children, the process of learning to eat, though seemingly effortless, is a complex task. At a physiologic level, feeding relies on two interrelated factors: structure and function. The basic physiologic complexity of feeding is further compounded by social and cultural aspects. Feeding development occurs in the context of a parent–child relationship within a larger family unit within a still larger culture. Thus, the development of feeding skills is a progression of physiologic tasks and behaviors which are gradually learned in a social context.

The purpose of this chapter is to describe the normal development of feeding in infants and young children. The chapter will begin with a description of the functional anatomy of the oral cavity and pharynx, followed by a discussion of the physiology and neurophysiology of infant and mature swallowing. The remainder of the chapter will discuss how children progress from infant feeding to mature eating and swallowing. A knowledge of normal feeding development, and the various factors affecting it, is essential to an understanding of feeding disorders in children with neurodevelopmental disabilities.

Functional anatomy of the mouth and pharynx

Structural integrity of the mouth and pharynx is necessary for normal feeding development (Fig. 2.1). Anatomically, the pharynx is made up of three compartments: the nasopharynx, the oropharynx, and the hypopharynx (Donner *et al.* 1985). The nasopharynx extends from the base of the skull to the roof of the soft palate. The oropharynx extends from the palate above to the base of the tongue below and includes the valleculae. The mouth, or oral cavity, is in continuity with the oropharynx. The hypopharynx extends from the valleculae to the cricopharyngeus, or upper esophageal sphincter. The larynx opens into the hypopharynx anteriorly via the laryngeal aditus (Donner *et al.* 1985). While the nasopharynx is not a part of the alimentary tract, the oropharynx and the hypopharynx are part of both the alimentary and respiratory tracts.

These anatomic compartments are involved in three categories of motor function: stabilization and maintenance of structural position and form, alimentation, and respiration (Bosma 1985). While these categories of function share common anatomic structures and motor units, each has its own network of neural control mechanisms and its own calendar of development (Bosma 1985). This chapter reviews only those functions related to alimentation.

Mature eating and swallowing has four phases: the oral-preparatory, oral, pharyngeal,

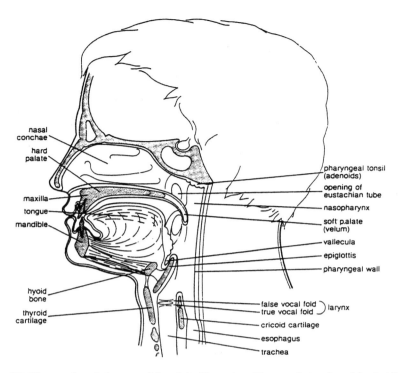

Fig. 2.1. The mouth and pharynx of the adult. (Reproduced by permission from Morris 1982.)

and esophageal phases. A total of 31 pairs of striated muscles are involved during the various phases of swallowing (Dodds *et al.* 1990). These muscles are important both as structural and functional elements. The muscles of the face, lips and mandible play an important role during the oral-preparatory phase. These muscles are innervated respectively by the facial nerve (VII) and the mandibular branch (V_3) of the trigeminal nerve. The tongue, which is important in both the oral-preparatory and the pharyngeal phases of swallowing, consists of four intrinsic and four extrinsic muscles. The intrinsic muscles are innervated by the hypoglossal nerve (XII), and the extrinsic muscles, with the exception of the palatoglossus (X) are innervated by the ansa cervicalis (C_1–C_2). Suprahyoid and infrahyoid muscle groups, responsible for hyoid and laryngeal movement, are innervated by V_3, VII and the ansa cervicalis (C_1–C_2). The muscles of the palate, pharynx and larynx, with few exceptions are innervated by the vagus (X).

Although the basic arrangement of the mouth, pharynx and larynx in the infant is similar to that of the adult, some differences are noteworthy (Fig. 2.2). The tongue, the soft palate, and the arytenoid mass (arytenoid cartilage, false vocal cords and true vocal cords) are large relative to their surrounding chambers when compared with the adult (Bosma 1985). In the infant, the tongue lies entirely within the oral cavity (Bosma 1985, Tuchman 1988). In addition, the lateral walls of the oral cavity are stabilized by a sucking pad, composed

12

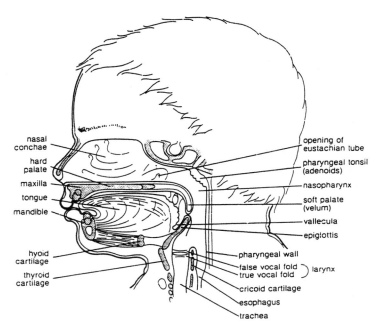

nasal conchae

hard palate

maxilla

tongue

mandible

hyoid cartilage

thyroid cartilage

opening of eustachian tube

pharyngeal tonsil (adenoids)

nasopharynx

soft palate (velum)

vallecula

epiglottis

pharyngeal wall

false vocal fold ⎫ larynx
true vocal fold ⎭

cricoid cartilage

esophagus

trachea

Fig. 2.2. The mouth and pharynx of the newborn infant. (Reproduced by permission from Morris 1982.)

of densely compacted fatty tissue, which results in a small oropharynx (Bosma 1986). The larynx lies high and anteriorly in the infant (Kramer and Eicher 1993), and the tip of the epiglottis extends to and may overlap the soft palate. This position of the epiglottis helps protect against aspiration by diverting the liquid diet laterally around the laryngeal opening. These anatomic relationships are ideal for the normal infant feeding pattern, suck/suckle feeding from a breast or a bottle in a recumbent position (Kramer 1989).

As the head and neck grow, the oral cavity enlarges about the tongue, the upper pharynx enlarges about the soft palate, and the laryngeal vestibule enlarges in relation to the arytenoid mass (Bosma 1985). The fat pads disappear, the neck elongates and the larynx descends gradually to its adult position. In addition, from 6 to 12 months postnatally, the dentition begins to erupt. The teeth add new structural units with both sensory and mechanical functions. The importance of the teeth in the acquisition of biting and chewing skills is difficult to assess. Bosma (1986) has suggested that the teeth may be more important as sensory organs and that their sensory inputs may be critical to the development of central control of feeding.

These anatomic relationships in the mouth and pharynx of the infant and young child change with physical growth. However, with the exception of tooth eruption and partial descent of the larynx within the pharynx, most of the anatomic changes begin in the third and fourth year (Bosma 1986), which is after the development of most feeding skills. Thus, maturation of feeding skills over the first few years of life, while influenced by the anatomic

13

TABLE 2.1
Feeding reflexes present in the newborn infant

Reflex	Stimulus	Response	Time of disappearance
Suck–swallow	Stroke anterior third of tongue or center of lips	Suckle/suck, swallow	4 months
Rooting	Stroke around the mouth	Move head toward source of stimulus, latch on to nipple	3–4 months (later if breast-fed)
Biting	Stroke the gum	Rhythmic up and down biting motions of the jaw	6 months
Gagging	Mid-third portion of tongue	Gag, eye widening	Moves to posterior third of tongue at 7 months
Babkin's	Stroke (firmly) the palms of both hands	Mouth opens, head flexes and rotates to midline	3–4 months

changes associated with growth, is accomplished largely by developmental changes in the central nervous system coupled with experiential learning. Nevertheless, normal feeding development depends on anatomic integrity. While the swallowing apparatus has some capacity to compensate for specific structural or functional deficits (Buchholz *et al.* 1985), it is clear that most anatomic abnormalities (*e.g.* cleft lip, tracheo-esophageal fistula) significantly affect feeding and swallowing.

Swallowing physiology
Infant sucking, swallowing and breathing
Feeding in the newborn infant differs from mature feeding (Bosma 1992). Mature feeding involves multiple methods of eating (*e.g.* spoon, cup, chewing) and manipulation of food in the oral cavity. Infant feeding involves a single method which intertwines sucking, swallowing and breathing. It is not possible to separate its components. In addition, the delivery of the food bolus into the pharynx of the infant differs in its rate and rhythm from the mature eating pattern, and mature feeding has more volitional components than infant feeding.

The newborn infant is reflex-bound and automatically makes certain oral movements (Table 2.1). For example, the rooting reflex, elicited by stroking the side of the mouth and resulting in the head turning toward the source of the stimulus, is a food-seeking response (Wolf and Glass 1992). When the nipple is drawn close to the mouth, the rooting reflex helps the baby latch onto the bottle or breast. Interpreting the presence, absence or diminution of an oral reflex must be done within the environmental context in which it occurs. Some reflexes, such as rooting or sucking, may depend on hunger or satiety, the state or level of alertness, or the infant's neurologic status (Wolf and Glass 1992).

Sucking
The muscles of the tongue, including the fan-like genioglossus, provide a peristaltic action

which compresses the nipple in a wavelike fashion and allows the infant to express liquid. The entire tongue, the mandible and the lower lip are moved in alternating phases downward and forward and upward and back. At birth, the infant's anatomic structure dictates that the tongue move in an extension–retraction pattern because of the limited room within the oral cavity. This initial in-and-out pattern is called suckling and resembles a lick-suck (Evans Morris and Klein 1987). A variation on this basic, reflexive suckle pattern is recognized as a true suck. In the true suck, the body or dorsum of the tongue moves up and down in conjunction with the mandible, the lips close more tightly around the nipple, and more negative pressure is created in the oral cavity to extract fluid. Most infants utilize a mixture of suck and suckle until 6 months of age. By 6 months the true suck predominates, as it is generally more efficient (Evans Morris and Klein 1987).

Swallowing
Moving the liquid bolus (milk) via the tongue from the front to the back of the oral cavity appears to be a continuous motion which begins with sucking. The swallow results when a sufficient amount of milk accumulates either in the back of the oral cavity or in the valleculae (Bosma 1992). During this stage the bolus is propelled not only by muscle action but also by the changing of pressure gradients throughout the mouth, pharynx and esophagus (Bosma 1992). The momentum of the bolus helps project it into the pharynx at a rapid rate.

Breathing
Respiratory rate is closely coordinated with swallowing and must be altered during feeding because of the obligatory periods of apnoea which occur with swallowing. These periods decrease the overall time available to breathe. During much of infant feeding the suck, swallow and breathe triad are stable in a 1:1:1 relation. Coordinated breathing in an expiration–inspiration pattern is a necessary requisite to successful feeding. During continuous sucking the overall respiratory rate decreases, the expiratory phase lengthens, and the inspiratory phase shortens. Intermittent sucking causes the respiratory rate to return to baseline (Wolf and Glass 1992).

Respiration patterns vary with infant age and development. The 1-month-old sequences two or more sucks from the breast or bottle before pausing to swallow and breathe (Evans Morris and Klein 1987). By 6 months the infant has learned to use longer and longer sequences of sucking, swallowing and breathing. Infants must cease respiration during the pharyngeal stage of swallow and are obligate nose breathers during feeding. Given their small oropharynx and the presence of a nipple they have no choice but to nose breathe. Since oxygen requirements take precedence over feeding requirements, infants with breathing difficulties of any kind do not feed well. Similarly, nasal obstructions can interfere with feeding.

Mature swallowing
The four phases of mature eating and swallowing are the oral-preparatory, oral, pharyngeal and esophageal phases (Table 2.2). The collection of food, liquid or saliva into a swallow-ready bolus requires preparation by the tongue, jaw, teeth, palate and lips (Loge-

TABLE 2.2
Mature swallowing behavior

Stage	Structures	Activities	Time
Oral preparation (voluntary)	Lips Tongue Cheeks Palate	Lips close Food mixed with saliva and masticated	Varies depending on substance
Phase I: Oral phase (voluntary/ involuntary)	Tongue	Moves bolus posteriorly Triggers swallow reflex at pharyngeal wall	Less than 1 second
Phase II: Pharyngeal phase (involuntary)	Velum Pharyngeal constrictor Epiglottis Laryngeal strap muscle Arytenoid mass Upper esophageal sphincter	Velum elevates Pharyngeal peristalsis Epiglottis closes Larynx closes, elevates and draws forward Upper esophageal sphincter relaxes	1 second or less
Phase III: Esophageal phase (involuntary)	Esophagus	Enters esophagus Moves to stomach	8–20 seconds

mann 1983, Evans Morris and Klein 1987, Fox 1990). Solid foods are lateralized by the tongue to the grinding surface of the teeth, masticated, mixed with saliva and drawn together into a bolus. Liquid or saliva does not require as much preparation but is collected or drawn together. After this preparation is complete, the three phases of swallowing begin. The tongue first creates a groove or trough and elevates and projects the bolus backward by using peristaltic action. When the bolus reaches the posterior oral cavity (*i.e.* the soft palate and faucial pillars) the swallow reflex is activated (Wolf and Glass 1992). This sensory stimulus on the posterior oral structures ends the voluntary oral phase and triggers the involuntary pharyngeal phase of swallow. During the pharyngeal phase, the velum elevates, closing off the nasopharynx, and the pharyngeal constrictors propel the bolus through the faucial pillars to the upper esophageal sphincter (cricopharyngeus) in a peristaltic wave. Concomitantly, the larynx closes, elevates, and is pulled forward by the laryngeal strap muscles. The epiglottis and the aryepiglottic folds, the false vocal folds, and the true vocal folds form three separate levels of laryngeal closure, protecting the airway from penetration by food or liquid. Respiration stops briefly to allow the bolus to move to the relaxed upper esophageal sphincter. The cricopharyngeus muscle serves as the valve at the top of the esophagus. It remains in a fixed state of contraction and only relaxes to allow food or liquid to pass during a swallow. The esophageal phase then begins and involves a continuation of peristaltic transport of the bolus to the stomach.

Neurophysiologic control of swallowing
Deglutition, or swallowing, is defined as the semiautomatic motor action of the muscles of the respiratory and gastrointestinal tracts to propel food from the oral cavity to the stomach

(Miller 1986). This motor action is stimulated and modified by sensory stimuli from the mouth, pharynx and larynx, as well as higher central nervous system stimuli. The physiology and neurophysiology of swallowing is quite complex. The neural control of swallowing involves four components: (1) afferent sensory fibers contained in four cranial nerves (V_3, VII, IX, X); (2) efferent motor fibers contained in five cranial nerves (V_3, VII, IX, X, XII) and two cervical peripheral nerves (C_1,C_2); (3) paired brainstem swallowing centers in the medulla; and (4) modifying neural input from the pons, the limbic–hypothalamic system, the cerebellum and the prefrontal cortex (Miller 1986, Dodds *et al.* 1990). The brainstem swallowing centers integrate and process various input signals from oropharyngeal sensory fibers and higher CNS centers and then orchestrate the swallowing process via efferent motor fibers in the cranial nerves.

Sensory nerve input to the medullary swallowing centers is provided mainly by cranial nerves IX and X with some input from the maxillary branch of the trigeminal (V_3) and facial (VII) nerves (Dodds *et al.* 1990). It is believed that coded sensory information of a specific pattern and intensity from a receptive field of the oral cavity, tongue and pharynx serves as the major trigger for swallowing (Ekberg and Hilderfors 1985, Dodds *et al.* 1990). The sensory pattern is believed to be critical for differentiating which motor response is evoked, as stimulation of the same anatomic region can evoke distinctly different motor responses (*e.g.* swallowing *versus* gagging or vomiting) (Miller 1982). Cortical input to the medullary centers, such as the conscious intent to swallow, are thought to facilitate oropharyngeal sensory stimuli (Dodds *et al.* 1990). Thus, such higher cortical factors probably influence the type of motor response elicited by sensory stimuli. In addition to triggering the reflexive swallow, local sensory mechanisms are believed to modulate or adapt the swallow depending on the size and characteristics of the bolus, head and neck posture at the time of the swallow, and orientation to gravity (Buchholz *et al.* 1985).

The medullary swallowing centers are more a functional system than a discrete anatomic locus, as they are not identifiable by neuron cell type or exact site (Donner *et al.* 1985). The swallowing centers consist of poorly defined areas comprising the nucleus tractus solitarius (NTS) and the ventro-medial reticular formation. Input sensory fibers from the cranial nerves and higher cerebral centers synapse within the NTS or reticular formation (Dodds *et al.* 1990). The neurons of the NTS then synapse with the primary motor nuclei in the nearby nucleus ambiguus (Bosma 1985). Each swallowing center consists of an elaborate array of interneurons which process incoming information from peripheral sensory fibers and higher cortical and subcortical centers and generate a preprogrammed swallowing response. This response is then delivered to the appropriate muscles via multiple cranial nerve motor nuclei and their corresponding axons (Dodds *et al.* 1990), resulting in a sequential activation–inactivation of muscle groups.

The neurophysiologic control of the oral-preparatory stage involves the volitional use of several craniofacial muscles (Miller 1982). Passage of the bolus to the posterior portion of the oral cavity initiates the involuntary pharyngeal phase with the concomitant inhibition of respiration. The pharyngeal stage consists of a rapid, stereotypic sequence of events (Miller 1982). The neurophysiologic control of this involuntary phase is currently best explained by the central pattern generator hypothesis with modification by peripheral feedback.

The central pattern generator hypothesis states that once swallowing is initiated, it is pre-programmed in a stereotypic manner by the medullary swallowing center. It is now believed that this programmed response can be modified by certain peripheral and cortical variables (Dodds et al. 1990).

Oral feeding for the newborn infant is entirely reflexive. Rooting, nipple latching, suck-ing and swallowing do not appear to require suprabulbar activity. Immediately after birth, however, the learning process begins with its dependence on experiential opportunities, sens-ory inputs and suprabulbar neurologic maturation. The whole process by which suprabulbar mechanisms become capable of utilizing the resources of the medullary swallowing centers to accomplish qualitatively different feeding tasks has been termed encephalization (Bosma 1986). Through feeding experience and the process of encephalization, different sensory inputs are extended past the brainstem to the midbrain, cerebellum, thalamus and cerebral cortex (Bosma 1986). These suprabulbar areas interpret the sensory input and exert their higher level of volitional control on the brainstem motor centers. As a result, the older infant and young child acquire the ability to evaluate the physical character of food, manipulate it appropriately, and voluntarily ingest it (Bosma 1986). It is of interest and rel-evance that children with athetoid cerebral palsy suppress oro-pharyngeal involuntary movements during swallowing. This illustrates the dominance of the movements involved in swallowing over other motor processes.

The learning of feeding skills

Eating and swallowing is such a natural, subconscious act that many adults forget that eating is a learned skill. Unlike breathing, which is similar to feeding in that it is largely subconscious with some element of voluntary control, most of feeding is learned behavior. While feeding begins as a reflex, it becomes a voluntary act with only the pharyngeal and esophageal parts of the swallow remaining under reflex control. Growth and neurologic maturation play a role in feeding development, but experiential learning is crucial. An im-portant aspect of learning is sensation and sensory feedback. This involves proprioception, touch, pressure, temperature and taste. Other important factors contributing to learning are gross and fine motor development, the methods of food presentation, and cognitive devel-opment. Finally, some believe that a 'critical period' exists for optimal learning of feeding skills.

Sensation and perception

The motor acts involved in feeding and swallowing are generally triggered by some sens-ory stimuli. It is not possible to directly quantify sensation, and information regarding normal sensory function in infants and young children is based on observation of behav-ioral responses to sensory stimuli (Evans Morris and Klein 1987). An infant's mouthing of his own hands and feet or of surrounding toys, furniture and other inanimate objects pro-vides needed experience for later feeding (Evans Morris and Klein 1987, Alexander 1991). This kind of exploration facilitates both motor and sensory development. For example, the gag reflex seen in the newborn infant is felt by some to modify itself within the first 6 months of life. That is, as an infant gains oral experience, the gag reflex recedes from the middle third of the tongue to the posterior third (Alexander 1991). Children with motor disabilities or medical problems which interfere with normal oral explorations may develop hypersensitivity to various kinds of sensory stimulation. They may gag when an empty spoon is placed on their tongue, cry during the feeding process, pull away as the spoon approaches because of unpleasant past associations, and refuse to try any new taste, texture, or method of feeding.

Related motor development and feeding

While feeding is primarily dependent on oral mechanisms, related motor development also plays a role. Gross motor development theory postulates that stability is needed before the infant can learn mobility (Evans Morris and Klein 1987). Head control and trunk stability provide the necessary gross motor foundation for the fine motor function seen in the hands and mouth. The oral motor movements needed in feeding occur after the head and trunk have achieved stability, symmetry and alignment.

Food is presented to children via bottle, spoon or cup. For the most part, these presentations are controlled by the feeder until children attain the eye–hand coordination which enables them to feed themselves. In order to finger-feed, for example, the child must acquire the upper extremity dexterity to progress to using a spoon and needs a transition food to progress from puréed food to hard solids. The integration of oral motor skills and self-feeding is mutually beneficial to each area of development.

Types of food

The types of food presented to young children represent culture, family preference, and individual likes and dislikes. Certain consistencies of food are by practice and convention felt to be easier to eat. However, the conventional practice of progressing from liquids to semi-solids or from puréed foods to solids must be recognized as a belief which is not supported by empirical data. Other cultures do not dwell on transitional feeding (*i.e.* puréed or easily chewed foods) but keep children on breast/bottle and wean to solid foods. This weaning depends on child factors (*e.g.* tooth eruption), maternal factors (*e.g.* pregnancy) and cultural weaning rules (Millard and Graham 1985).

New methods of food presentation cause children to revert to earlier patterns of oral motor skill. For example, when first given a spoonful of puréed food, a child uses a suckle pattern to extract the food. When given a bite of cracker, the child uses the same movement, the suckle, to chew the food. If presented with a hard-to-bite substance such as a thick pretzel stick, the child will suck or suckle it. With experience children learn to manipulate different types of food substances in qualitatively different ways.

Cognitive development and eating behaviors

Cognitive development, including language and non-verbal problem solving, plays a crucial role in the development of eating behaviors. Eating, like language, is acquired in the context of a responsive environment. It can be described in terms of the antecedent stimulus (S) which sets the occasion for a response (R) to occur, which, in turn, evokes other stimulus consequences (S^r) as follows (Siegel 1972): $S \rightarrow \rightarrow \rightarrow R \rightarrow \rightarrow \rightarrow S^r$.

This basic scheme offers a useful way to conceptualize how children learn to eat. The primary variables are the child, the stimulation she* receives (the food and the way it is presented) and the reinforcement her behaviour generates. Types of reinforcement include social and verbal praise provided by the caregiver, the pleasant feeling of satiation, and the interesting and appetizing taste of the food.

The caregiver's response to feeding behaviors is important to the child's development of competent feeding (Satter 1987). Mismanagement of the behaviors can confuse the child, and conversely the child's responses can confuse the caregiver. When certain physical reactions of the child interfere with feeding, the experience can become a negative one. For example, the feeling of satiety spoiled by gastric upset may become a negative and unpleasant reinforcement to oral feedings. The individual perceptions of taste, temperature and tactile input may also sway the child's responses in a contrary way. Children learn to associate certain events with eating and may generalize a few unpleasant experiences of eating to all other experiences.

Caregivers in the feeding relationship view their role as providing nourishment for their child. Their management of the child's behavioral responses to eating influences the child's subsequent assimilation of the feeding experience (Satter 1986, 1987). For example, if the caregiver responds with anxious and dogged persistence to mealtimes, prolongs the length of the meal, disregards the child's protests, and continues presenting food, the child may respond by refusing to eat at all. The child may learn to associate eating with confrontational negative experiences.

Communication is an important aspect of the feeding relationship. The communication is both verbal and nonverbal and involves expression and comprehension of hunger–satiety cues, food preferences and behavioral preferences. Nonverbal problem solving is also an important element of learning to eat through the child's persistent trial-and-error, cause-and-effect approach to mealtime. Fraiberg's notion of the 'little scientist' (Fraiberg 1959) is a fitting depiction of the toddler's task. In this context, the toddler also importantly begins to exert her will on her environment. The drive toward independence and mastery is often manifested quite strongly at the dinner table.

Concept of a critical period
The concepts of 'critical period' and 'sensitive period' are relevant to feeding development. A critical period refers to a fairly well delineated period of time during which a specific stimulus must be applied in order to produce a particular action. After such a critical period a particular behaviour pattern can no longer be learned (Illingworth and Lister 1964). The sensitive period refers to the optimal time for the application of a stimulus. After the sensitive period it is more difficult to learn a specific pattern of behaviour (Illingworth and Lister 1964). These concepts have been very well studied and described in animals, but have not been extensively studied in humans. They offer an attractive explanation for some feeding problems encountered in children. Preterm infants and those with severe gastrointestinal disease or central nervous system dysfunction may require prolonged enteral or

*The female pronoun is used for convenience throughout to represent both male and female children and adults.

20

parenteral feeding and thus be deprived of oral stimulation for a prolonged period of time. These children may be resistant to oral feedings and have great difficulty learning to eat (Blackman and Nelson 1987, Tuchman 1988).

Summary and conclusions

The development of feeding skills is a complex process which is influenced by multiple factors. The entire process depends on anatomic integrity. It begins in infants as the reflexive suckle–swallow–breathe triad at the bottle or breast. Gradually, through the process of encephalization and experience, children learn to ingest voluntarily a multitude of different foods. The learning of feeding skills takes place in the context of a close social relationship which plays an important role in the process. Most children negotiate the necessary developmental sequence without significant difficulty. Feeding disorders develop when the normal process is disrupted by various anatomic, neurologic, physiologic, psychologic and social factors. An understanding of the development of normal feeding provides an essential framework for the rational conceptualization, evaluation and management of children with developmental disabilities and feeding disorders.

ACKNOWLEDGEMENTS

The authors are grateful to Brenda M. Koonce, CPS, for her invaluable assistance with the manuscript. This work is supported, in part, by the Kluge Research Fund of the University of Virginia.

REFERENCES

Alexander, R. (1991) 'Prespeech and feeding.' *In:* Bigge, J.L. (Ed.) *Teaching Individuals with Physical and Multiple Disabilities.* New York: Macmillan, pp. 175–215.

Blackman, J.A., Nelson, C.L.A. (1987) 'Rapid introduction of oral feedings to tube-fed patients.' *Journal of Developmental and Behavioral Pediatrics*, **8**, 63–67.

Bosma, J.F. (1985) 'Postnatal ontogeny of performances of the pharynx, larynx, and mouth.' *American Review of Respiratory Disease*, **131**, S10–S15.

—— (1986) 'Development of feeding.' *Clinical Nutrition*, **5**, 210–218.

—— (1992) 'Pharyngeal swallow: basic mechanisms, development and impairments.' *Advances in Otolaryngology Head and Neck Surgery*, **6**, 225–275.

Buchholz, D.W., Bosma, J.F., Donner, M.W. (1985) 'Adaptation, compensation and decompensation of the pharyngeal swallow.' *Gastrointestinal Radiology*, **10**, 235–239.

Dodds, W.J., Stewart, E.T., Logemann, J.A. (1990) 'Physiology and radiology of the normal oral and pharyngeal phases of swallowing.' *American Journal of Roentgenology*, **154**, 953–963.

Donner, M.W., Bosma, J.F., Robertson, D.L. (1985) 'Anatomy and physiology of the pharynx.' *Gastrointestinal Radiology*, **10**, 196–212.

Ekberg, O., Hilderfors, H. (1985) 'Defective closure of the laryngeal vestibule: frequency of pulmonary complications.' *American Journal of Roentgenology*, **145**, 1159–1164.

Evans Morris, S., Klein, M.D. (1987) *Pre-feeding Skills: a Comprehensive Resource for Feeding Development.* Tucson, AZ: Therapy Skill Builders.

Fox, C.A. (1990) 'Implementing the modified barium swallow evaluation in children who have multiple disabilities.' *Infants and Young Children*, **3**, 67–77.

Fraiberg, S.H. (1959) *The Magic Years: Understanding and Handling the Problems of Early Childhood.* New York: Charles Scribner's Sons.

Illingworth, R.S., Lister, J. (1964) 'The critical or sensitive period, with special reference to certain feeding problems in infants and children.' *Journal of Pediatrics*, **65**, 839–848.

Kramer, S.S. (1989) 'Radiologic examination of the swallowing impaired child.' *Dysphagia*, **3**, 117–125.
—— Eicher, P.M. (1993) 'The evaluation of pediatric feeding abnormalities.' *Dysphagia*, **8**, 215–224.
Logemann, J. (1983) *Evaluation and Treatment of Swallowing Disorders.* San Diego: College Hill Press.
Millard, C.L., Graham, M.A. (1985) 'Breastfeed in two Mexican villages: social and demographic perspectives.' *In:* Hull, V. Simpson, M. (Eds.) *Breastfeeding, Child Health and Child Spacing: Cross-cultural Perspectives.* London: Croom Helm, pp. 55–61.
Miller, A.J. (1982) 'Deglutition.' *Physiological Reviews*, **62**, 129–184.
—— (1986) 'Neurophysiological basis of swallowing.' *Dysphagia*, **1**, 91–100.
Morris, S.E. (1982) *The Normal Acquisition of Oral Feeding Skills: Implications for Assessment and Treatment.* New York: Therapeutic Media.
Satter, E.M. (1986) 'The feeding relationship.' *Journal of the American Dietetic Association*, **86**, 352–356.
—— (1987) *How to Get Your Kid to Eat . . . But Not Too Much.* Palo Alto, CA: Bull Publishing Company.
Siegel, G.M. (1972) 'Three approaches to speech retardation.' *In:* Schiefelbusch, R.L. (Ed.) *Language of the Mentally Retarded.* Baltimore: University Park Press, pp. 127–143.
Tuchman, D.N. (1988) 'Dysfunctional swallowing in the pediatric patient: clinical considerations.' *Dysphagia*, **2**, 203–208.
Wolf, L.S., Glass, R.P. (1992) *Feeding and Swallowing Disorders in Infancy: Assessment and Management.* Tucson, AZ: Therapy Skill Builders.

3
THE CAUSES OF FEEDING DIFFICULTIES IN DISABLED CHILDREN

Peter B. Sullivan and Lewis Rosenbloom

As discussed in the previous chapter, feeding in the normal child is characterized by a progression from reflex-effected suckling followed at around 4 months by the gradual introduction of puréed and later solid and lumpy foods (transitional feeding) until finally, at about 24–30 months, the child is a relatively skilled tool user and can feed completely independently. The development of hand-regard from about 3 months of age is a component of integrating upper limb function into the infant's body image and is a prelude to using visually directed manual assistance in feeding; at 5 months the infant will start to hold the feeding bottle with both hands, at 6 months she will reach out and grasp a rusk, but not until about 8 or 9 months will she be able to finger feed effectively. At about this time, the child begins to understand that the spoon and the food go together and may even guide her mother's hand during feeding. At around 15 months the child is able to grasp the spoon and self-feed, albeit rather clumsily (Mueller 1975).

This natural progression does not happen in children who have cerebral palsy or other neurological disorders, for several possible reasons. These are detailed in Table 3.1. The various causes and pathology of neurological disability will not be described in this volume. The underlying neuropathology of oral-motor dysfunction is a degree of pseudobulbar palsy or of bulbar palsy and these may coexist in individual children. They may have a prenatal, perinatal or postnatal origin.

Failure of normal development of feeding ability and inadequate intake of calories may lead to undernutrition; up to 20 per cent of all disabled children may have an inadequate intake of food (Thommessen *et al.* 1991). Micronutrient deficiencies (with the exception of iron) are encountered less frequently in this group of children when compared with malnourished children in the developing world where both quantity and quality of diet are poor. Similarly, the loss of lean muscle mass in disabled children is probably related more to immobility than to inadequate protein intake. Malnutrition in disabled children, therefore, is largely a function of an insufficient amount of food being consumed rather than poor quality of food offered. This is not invariable, however, and in non-ambulatory disabled children without significant oral-motor dysfunction, obesity may become a serious handicap both for them and for their caretakers.

Although many individuals exhibit more than one disability, the primary cause of inadequate calorie intake in disabled children is slowness and inefficiency in feeding. Feeding efficiencies of less than 10 per cent are usual in severely disabled children (Ottenbacher *et al.* 1981, Gisel and Patrick 1988), from which it follows, as Patrick and Gisel (1990)

TABLE 3.1	TABLE 3.2
Causes of feeding difficulties in disabled children	**Common oral-motor deficits in a disabled child**
Oral-motor dysfunction	Poorly coordinated breathing
Disruption of the sensitive learning period	Choking
Dystonia	Difficulties with sucking and swallowing
Postural deformity	Persistence of the bite reflex
Impairment of hand function	Tonic biting
Immobility	Jaw instability
Visual impairment	Jaw thrusting
Deafness	Tongue thrusting
Gastro-oesophageal reflux	Decreased tongue movements
Recurrent aspiration	Failure of tongue lateralization
Dental problems	Poor lip closure
Constipation	Lip retraction
Communication difficulties	Drooling
Behavioural problems	Hypo- or hypersensitive gag response

observe, that up to 10 times the normal daily feeding time would be required to support a normal body and a normal metabolism. While prolonged feeding times may compensate for feeding inefficiency when the disabled child is small, as body size increases a point is reached at which no further compensation is possible and growth is limited by energy intake. Nevertheless, in contrast to reports that mothers of disabled children spend prolonged periods of time feeding (Johnson and Deitz 1985, Gisel and Patrick 1988), Reilly and Skuse, who assessed 12 infants with moderate to severe oral-motor dysfunction and marked failure to thrive, found that their mean duration of meal times did not differ from that of controls. The dietary intakes of two groups of subjects, however, did differ significantly, as the disabled children were both offered and consumed less food (Reilly and Skuse 1992). This observation of inadequate amounts of food being presented possibly reflects the situation for the majority of disabled children. It is particularly true for children living in institutions with a low caretaker-to-patient ratio where there is insufficient time to properly assist inefficient feeders.

Any of the factors listed in Table 3.1 can contribute to inefficiency in feeding and growth impairment. These will be discussed in more detail.

Oral-motor dysfunction

Predictable deficits are commonly associated with abnormal oral-motor development (Table 3.2). The relationship between oral-motor dysfunction and growth retardation has been clearly documented by Krick and Van Duyn (1984). In their study, children with cerebral palsy and oral-motor difficulties were found to be significantly thinner by age and height than their age- and sex-matched counterparts with cerebral palsy but no oral-motor impairment.

Oral neuromotor reflexes such as rooting, suckle feeding, gagging and biting are present at birth and gradually mature so that by 3 years of age they are similar to adult patterns. Graduation from suckle feeding to transitional feeding occurs mainly as a result of central nervous system maturation (Bosma 1986). Sensory stimulation is important in influencing the central processing that initiates the patterned sequence of movements common to functional oral activities. Oral-motor deficits are associated with both sensory and motor dysfunction. Persistence of primitive oral reflexes will delay the development of mature oral-motor function (Hargrove 1980, McBride and Danner 1987).

Mature feeding patterns are characterized by coordinated breathing and swallowing, rotary chewing, and precise tongue and lip movements which permit sucking and swallowing to occur with minimal jaw movement so that all textures of food may be eaten. Disabled children frequently spill much of the food offered to them. Korabek and colleagues (1981) estimated that as much as 11 per cent of all food offered to the profoundly disabled children in their study was lost in spillage. Patrick and Gisel (1990) have observed that if spillage is a problem, a good response to conventional treatment is unlikely.

Neurologically impaired children also have difficulty with the initiation of chewing. Hence, the delay from placement of food in the mouth until the onset of chewing may be a sensitive indicator of feeding impairment (Stolovitz and Gisel 1991). The lips and cheeks participate more definitely in the eating process during infancy than in adults (Gisel 1991). Moreover, eating with the mouth open may be the preferred strategy in younger children who must coordinate breathing and swallowing and, as McPherson and colleagues (1992) note, such co-ordination is less necessary when chewing solids.

Dental problems

Promoting the dental health of disabled children is an important component of multidisciplinary care. Dental caries, peri-odontal disease and gingival hyperplasia can all contribute to feeding difficulties in their own right. Secondary orthodontic problems such as the presence of malocclusion, overjet and overbite occur as a consequence of oral-motor maldevelopment and again exacerbate feeding problems.

Disruption of the sensitive learning period

Introduction of solid foods to the diet of an infant is most important both for diminution in the strength of the gag response and for the development of more active tongue, jaw and cheek/lip movements in chewing activities. Several authors have suggested that there is a 'critical' or 'sensitive' period with respect to the development of normal feeding patterns (Illingworth and Lister 1964, Blackman and Nelson 1985, Geertsma et al. 1985). The ability to handle solid foods is usually evident at 6 months of age. Younger children display more mature feeding behaviours when presented with solid rather than softer textures. Note, however, that they often revert to suckling behaviour with purées, whereas chewing motions are used with solids. Eating solid foods requires that the tongue works independently of the jaw and, by so doing, supports the more mature feeding behaviour (Stolovitz and Gisel 1991). Many disabled children, however, persist in eating puréed foods long past the age when most children begin to eat textured and lumpy foods. This is often because it is the only type of food which their caretaker can get them to take. Delayed introduction of solids and prolonged subsistence on puréed foods was found to be due to neuromotor dysfunction in 79 per cent cases studied by Palmer and colleagues (1975), while most of the remainder were secondary to behavioural problems of one sort or another. This dependence on puréed foods not only impairs the normal development of oral-motor function but also potentially limits total calorie intake due to dilution and early satiety and, because it is low in dietary fibre, contributes to constipation in the disabled (Fischer et al.1985).

Gastrointestinal dysfunction

There are more neurons in the enteric nervous system than in the spinal cord (Menkes and Ament 1988). It is then not surprising that insults to the central nervous system may result in significant dysfunction in the gastrointestinal tract. In addition to the dysphagia described above, rumination, cricopharyngeal achalasia, gastro-oesophageal reflux, with or without aspiration, delayed gastric emptying and constipation are all potential problems which can contribute to feeding difficulty in disabled children. These and other disorders reflect abnormalities of bowel motility.

Rumination, which is the frequent regurgitation of previously ingested food into the mouth where it is chewed, is common in disabled children and can occur at any time during, following or long after eating (Schärli 1985). Schärli reported four children with severe mental retardation who were malnourished secondary to vomiting in association with rumination.

Gastro-oesophageal reflux (GOR) contributes significantly to dysphagia (Catto-Smith et al. 1991) and is relatively common in disabled children; up to 75 per cent of children with cerebral palsy have been shown to have GOR in some series (Abrahams and Burkitt 1970, Sondheimer and Morris 1979, Reyes et al. 1993). In both developmentally delayed and normal infants with chronic GOR, resistance to eating sufficient to cause failure to thrive has been demonstrated (Byrne et al. 1982, Dellert et al. 1993). The majority of children with histologically proven oesophagitis have GOR (Baer et al. 1986), and pain from reflux oesophagitis can inhibit eating. Discomfort from GOR may account for irritability in disabled children, and this diagnosis is frequently overlooked because of their inability to communicate. Unusual posturing, Sandifer's syndrome, is a rare but well-defined manifestation of GOR. This syndrome, which also includes iron deficiency anaemia and severe oesophagitis, was first described by Kinsbourne in 1964. It is usually seen in infants and young children and manifests as peculiar head-cocking movements that characteristically involve extension of the neck and rotation of the head, usually during or immediately after meals (Herbst 1981). It has been suggested that the abnormal movements are involuntarily controlled attempts to prevent reflux and relieve pain. In normal children these movements usually prompt extensive psychological evaluation which can delay the diagnosis of GOR, while in disabled children the syndrome is likely to be attributed to an associated movement disorder.

Recurrent aspiration pneumonia will impair feeding ability and is a further potential complication of chronic GOR which has been widely reported (Cadman et al. 1978, Euler et al. 1979, Berquist et al. 1981, Byrne et al. 1982, Fung et al. 1990). About 50 per cent of children with GOR will also have delayed gastric emptying (DGE) (Campbell et al. 1989). The association between GOR and DGE has been demonstrated in both normal (Hillemeier et al. 1983, Papaila et al. 1989) children and those with disorders of the central nervous system (Fonkalsrud et al. 1992). This association, however, may to some extent depend on the type of food given (Jolley *et al.* 1987, Fried *et al.* 1992, Heacock *et al.* 1992, Sutphen and Dillard 1992, Tolia *et al.* 1992). Nevertheless, as Van Winckel and Robbe-recht (1993) observe, trying to treat GOR without effectively treating DGE may be one of the reasons why treatment, both conservative and surgical, of GOR in profoundly disabled children gives such poor results (Pearl *et al.* 1990, Smith *et al.* 1992, Rogers *et al.* 1993).

Constipation and faecal impaction are significant and common problems in non-ambulatory, neurologically impaired children (Webb 1980). Although little is known about the precise pathophysiology of bowel function of children with severe disabilities, it is readily apparent from the prevalence of constipation and the regular use of elimination aids in this population that bowel function is abnormal (Fischer *et al.* 1985). The possibility exists that there is an underlying defect in gut innervation. The problem is exacerbated by medica-tion, physical inactivity and the use of puréed foods. Constipation is associated with early satiety and is an additional reason for poor feeding in disabled children; it was found to be a contributory factor to undernutrition in 41 per cent of cases in one series (Pesce *et al.* 1989).

Associated neurological problems
Other manifestations of static encephalopathies occur very commonly in children with cerebral palsy. These include epilepsy, visual impairment, learning difficulties ranging in severity from mild to profound, and emotional and behavioural disorders. All of these may contribute to and exacerbate feeding difficulties. Postural deformity, impairment of hand function, dystonia and tactile hypersensitivity, all problems associated with central neuro-logical damage, can also adversely influence feeding ability.

Dystonia and tactile hypersensitivity
The oral-motor deficits found in disabled children occur in the context of central neuro-logical damage and are frequently associated with other forms of sensory or motor dys-function. Tactile hypersensitivity and muscular dystonia, for instance, commonly coexist with oral-motor dysfunction in disabled children. Children with hypotonia, for instance, are often unable to stabilize their heads and trunks, which can impair their ability to initiate or sustain sucking, swallowing, biting or chewing (Ottenbacher *et al.* 1983). In contrast, those with hypertonus often demonstrate strong extensor patterns of the head, trunk and limbs. These limit oral movements which frequently become stereotyped and abnormal, with jaw and tongue thrusting together with lip retraction. Such stereotyped patterns pre-clude mouth closure, fine tongue movements, coordinated chewing and swallowing, and result in drooling, loss of food and choking (Ottenbacher *et al.* 1983). Tactile hypersensi-tivity may be most marked around the mouth, and disabled children may abreact so strongly to face washing or tooth brushing as to evoke generalized hypertonus or opisthotonos. As Mueller (1972) notes, oral tactile hypersensitivity is always followed by feeding problems as the child reacts to each stimulation of the spoon, cup, food or liquid in her mouth. Per-sistent oral reflexes tend to be the primary response to tactile stimulation in the child with oral and facial hypersensitivity (Morris 1989) and as long as these reflexes persist, feeding and early speech patterns are disrupted (Ottenbacher *et al.* 1983).

Postural deformity

Several associated sequelae of neuromotor dysfunction contribute to the feeding problems in disabled children. The athetoid child and the severely spastic quadriplegic child are often unable to sustain control of their head and trunk. This lack of sitting balance coupled with contractural deformity, inability to bend the hips sufficiently to reach forward to grasp, and failure to maintain that grasp irrespective of the position of the arms pose considerable problems for successful feeding. Moreover, inability to bring the hands to the mouth and lack of eye–hand coordination together with impairment of hand function render self-feeding a virtual impossibility for some children. Immobility also potentially contributes to the feeding problems of non-ambulatory disabled children who are unable to forage for food and, therefore, are completely dependant on others to bring them food. Attention to posture, including the provision of appropriate seating, is therefore a fundamental prerequisite to safe and effective feeding of severely disabled children.

Drug therapy

Drugs used in the management of cerebral palsy and associated conditions may have an additional adverse effect on feeding and nutritional status. A number of agents are used to reduce spasticity, for example baclofen, diazepam, botulinum toxin and dantrolene. All may produce some degree of unwanted hypotonia with adverse effects on posture and oral-motor function. In addition, baclofen and diazepam have the potential for more generalized sedation as do other sedatives, for example chloral hydrate and trimeprazine. These are sometimes prescribed for sleeping difficulties or irritability and their use can be counterproductive if a consequence is decreased alertness at mealtimes.

Anticonvulsants may also have a similar sedative effect, notably the benzodiazepines, carbamazepine and phenobarbitone, while in general all anticonvulsant drugs appear to have the potential in some children to cause anorexia and vomiting. By contrast, sodium valproate may act as an appetite stimulant and excessive weight gain is seen in a minority of treated children. Phenytoin has the particular disadvantage of gingival hyperplasia and hence commonly adversely effects dental hygiene and impairs chewing. Again, phenytoin (and phenobarbitone when it is used) may precipitate deficiencies in serum folate and abnormalities in vitamin D and bone metabolism (Crosley *et al.* 1975, Tolman *et al.* 1975). Other drugs used in disabled children may diminish appetite including tranquillizers and methlyphenidate. Tricyclic antidepressants also have anticholinergic properties and can impair eating ability as a result of xerostomia.

Some profoundly disabled children including many who are tube-fed are prescribed multiple medications, for example for spasticity, epilepsy, GOR, constipation and vitamin deficiency. These together make up a very significant volume that has to be administered several times daily. This can have a satiating effect upon their appetite and can contribute to nutritional failure. It is essential, therefore, that disabled children should have their drug regimens critically reviewed at regular intervals with attention paid to the necessity for each medication, the timing and administration of medications, side-effects, the possibility of drug interactions, and the consistency and volumes of the preparations prescribed. Non-prescribed medications that are being administered should also be ascertained.

Visual impairment

From birth, vision plays an important part in the feeding process. Norris and colleagues (1957) reported that it was only by 3 years of age that more than half of their large sample of blind children could manage to eat unassisted with a spoon, an ability that is expected to appear in the second year in sighted children. Visual impairment is a frequent concomitant of neurological disability in childhood (Jan 1993), and significant numbers of children with cerebral palsy and severe learning difficulties have little or no useful sight (Kitzinger 1980). Under such circumstances the co-ordinating role of vision is lost and the acquisition of feeding abilities is significantly prejudiced. The particular developmental pathways of visually impaired children, including their acquisition of social skills, necessitate the use of specific assessment methods, for example the Reynell–Zinkin Scales (Reynell 1979). Sonksen (1993) has described the principles of how relevant developmental help including the promotion of communication and feeding skills can be offered to young children with multiple disabilities and visual impairment.

Behavioural problems

Emotional disorders and behavioural problems have a significantly increased prevalence in children with neurological disorders (Rutter *et al.* 1970), and feeding difficulty is a frequent manifestation. Again autistic behavioural features with or without accompanying mental retardation can hinder normal feeding and lead to inadequate dietary intake. Chronic food refusal, therefore, can and has been shown to contribute to undernutrition in disabled children (Riordan *et al.* 1984). Fears and avoidance reactions are not uncommonly encountered in disabled children in relation to food. To compound these problems there can be frustration in the child with communication difficulty who cannot express hunger or food preferences, and frustration in the caretaker who cannot interpret the cues from the child. Palmer and Horn (1978) concluded that behavioural mismanagement was the primary factor associated with over 21 per cent of all feeding problems in disabled children referred to their nutrition clinic over a four year period. In another report on nutritional problems in disabled children (Pesce *et al.* 1989) behavioural problems were identified as contributory factors in 52 per cent of cases. Palmer and colleagues (1975) identified behavioural mismanagement as a contributor to the prolonged subsistence of their group of children on puréed foods. These authors, however, stressed the multifactorial nature of feeding problems in disabled children and the need for a multidisciplinary approach to management.

REFERENCES

Abrahams, P., Burkitt, B.F. (1970) 'Hiatus hernia and gastro-oesophageal reflux in children and adolescents with cerebral palsy.' *Australian Paediatric Journal*, **6**, 41–46.

Baer, M., Mäki, M., Nurminen, J., Turjanmaa, V., Pukander, J., Vesikari, T. (1986) 'Esophagitis and findings of long-term esophageal pH recording in children with repeated lower respiratory tract symptoms.' *Journal of Pediatric Gastroenterology and Nutrition*, **5**, 187–190.

Berquist, W.E., Rachelefsky, G.S., Kadden, M., Siegel, S.C., Katz, R.M., Fonkalsrud, E.W., Ament, M.E. (1981) 'Gastroesophageal reflux-associated recurrent pneumonia and chronic asthma in children.' *Pediatrics*, **68**, 29–35.

Blackman, J.A., Nelson, C.L.A. (1985) 'Reinstituting oral feedings in children fed by gastrostomy tube.' *Clinical Pediatrics*, **24**, 434–438.

Bosma, J.F. (1986) 'Development of feeding.' *Clinical Nutrition*, **5**, 210–218.

Byrne, W.J., Euler, A.R., Ashcraft, E., Nash, D.G., Seibert, J.J., Golladay, E.S. (1982) 'Gastroesophageal reflux in the severely retarded who vomit: criteria for and results of surgical intervention in twenty-two patients.' *Surgery*, **91**, 95–98.

Cadman, D., Richards, J., Feldman, W. (1978) 'Gastro-esophageal reflux in severely retarded children.' *Developmental Medicine and Child Neurology*, **20**, 95–98.

Campbell, J.R., Gilchrist, B.F., Harrison, M.W. (1989) 'Pyloroplasty in association with Nissen fundoplication in children with neurologic disorders.' *Journal of Pediatric Surgery*, **24**, 375–377.

Catto-Smith, A.G., Machida, H., Butzner, J.D., Gall, D.G., Scott, R.B. (1991) 'The role of gastroesophageal reflux in pediatric dysphagia.' *Journal of Pediatric Gastroenterology and Nutrition*, **12**, 159–165.

Crosley, C.J., Chee, C., Berman, P.H. (1975) 'Rickets associated with long-term anticonvulsant therapy in a pediatric outpatient population.' *Pediatrics*, **56**, 52–57.

Dellert, S.F., Hyams, J.S., Treem, W.R., Geertsma, M.A. (1993) 'Feeding resistance and gastroesophageal reflux in infancy.' *Journal of Pediatric Gastroenterology and Nutrition*, **17**, 66–71.

Euler, A.R., Byrne, W.J., Ament, M.E., Fonkalsrud, E.W., Strobel, C.T., Siegel, S.C., Katz, R.M., Rachelefsky, G.S. (1979) 'Recurrent pulmonary disease in children: a complication of gastroesophageal reflux.' *Pediatrics*, **63**, 47–51.

Fischer, M., Adkins, W., Hall, L., Scaman, P., Hsi, S., Marlett, J. (1985) 'The effects of dietary fibre in a liquid diet on bowel function of mentally retarded individuals.' *Journal of Mental Deficiency Research*, **29**, 373–381.

Fonkalsrud, E.W., Ament, M.E., Vargas, J. (1992) 'Gastric antroplasty for the treatment of delayed gastric emptying and gastroesophageal reflux in children.' *American Journal of Surgery*, **164**, 327–331.

Fried, M.D., Khoshoo, V., Secker, D.J., Gilday, D.L., Ash, J.M., Pencharz, P.B. (1992) 'Decrease in gastric emptying time and episodes of regurgitation in children with spastic quadriplegia fed a whey-based formula.' *Journal of Pediatrics*, **120**, 569–572.

Fung, K.P., Seagram, G., Pasieka, J., Trevenen, C., Machida, H., Scott, B. (1990) 'Investigation and outcome of 121 infants and children requiring Nissen fundoplication for the management of gastroesophageal reflux.' *Clinical and Investigative Medicine*, **13**, 237–246.

Geertsma, M.A., Hyams, J.S., Pelletier, J.M.,Reiter, S. (1985) 'Feeding resistance after parenteral hyperalimentation.' *American Journal of Diseases of Children*, **139**, 255–256.

Gisel, E.G. (1991) 'Effect of food texture on the development of chewing of children between six months and two years of age.' *Developmental Medicine and Child Neurology*, **33**, 69–79.

—— Patrick, J. (1988) 'Identification of children with cerebral palsy unable to maintain a normal nutritional state.' *Lancet*, **1**, 283–286.

Hargrove, R. (1980) 'Feeding the severely dysphagic patient.' *Journal of Neurosurgical Nursing*, **12**, 102–107.

Heacock, H.J., Jeffery, H.E., Baker, J.L., Page, M. (1992) 'Influence of breast versus formula milk on physiological gastroesophageal reflux in healthy, newborn infants.' *Journal of Pediatric Gastroenterology and Nutrition*, **14**, 41–46.

Herbst, J.J. (1981) 'Gastroesophageal reflux.' *Journal of Pediatrics*, **98**, 859–870.

Hillemeier, A.C., Grill, B.B., McCallum, R., Gryboski, J. (1983) 'Esophageal and gastric motor abnormalities in gastroesophageal reflux during infancy.' *Gastroenterology*, **84**, 741–746.

Illingworth, R.S., Lister, J. (1964) 'The critical or sensitive period, with special reference to certain feeding problems in infants and children.' *Journal of Pediatrics*, **65**, 839–848.

Jan, J.E. (1993) 'Neurological causes and investigation.' *In:* Fielder, A.R., Best, A.B., Bax, M.C.O. (Eds.) *The Management of Visual Impairment in Childhood. Clinics in Developmental Medicine No. 128.* London: Mac Keith Press, pp. 48–63.

Johnson, C.B., Deitz, J.C. (1985) 'Time use of mothers with preschool children: a pilot study.' *American Journal of Occupational Therapy*, **39**, 578–583.

Jolley, S.G., Leonard, J.C., Tunell, W.P. (1987) 'Gastric emptying in children with gastroesophageal reflux. I. An estimate of effective gastric emptying.' *Journal of Pediatric Surgery*, **22**, 923–926.

Kinsbourne, M. (1964) 'Hiatus hernia with contortions of the neck.' *Lancet*, **1**, 1058–1061.

Kitzinger, M. (1980) 'Planning management of feeding in the visually handicapped child.' *Child: Care, Health, and Development*, **6**, 291–299.

Korabek, C.A., Reid, D.H., Ivancic, M.T. (1981) 'Improving needed food intake of profoundly handicapped children through effective supervision of institutional staff.' *Applied Research in Mental Retardation*, **2**, 69–88.

Krick, J., Van Duyn, M.A.S. (1984) 'The relationship between oral-motor involvement and growth: a pilot study in a pediatric population with cerebral palsy.' *Journal of the American Dietetic Association*, **84**, 555–559.

McBride, M.C., Danner, S.C. (1987) 'Sucking disorders in neurologically impaired infants: assessment and facilitation of breastfeeding.' *Clinics in Perinatology*, **14**, 109–130.

McPherson, K.A., Kenny, D.J., Koheil, R., Bablich, K., Sochaniwskyj, A., Milner, M. (1992) 'Ventilation and swallowing interactions of normal children and children with cerebral palsy.' *Developmental Medicine and Child Neurology*, **34**, 577–588.

Menkes, J.H., Ament, M.E. (1988) 'Neurologic disorders of gastroesophageal function.' *Advances in Neurology*, **49**, 409–416.

Morris, S.E. (1989) 'Development of oral-motor skills in the neurologically impaired child receiving non-oral feedings.' *Dysphagia*, **3**, 135–154.

Mueller, H. (1975) 'Feeding.' *In:* Finnie, N.R. (Ed.) *Handling the Young Cerebral Palsied Child at Home.* New York: E.P. Dutton, pp. 113–132.

Norris, M., Spaulding, P.J., Brodie, F.H. (1957) *Blindness in Children.* Chicago: University of Chicago Press.

Ottenbacher, K., Scoggins, A., Wayland, J. (1981) 'The effectiveness of a program of oral sensory motor therapy with the severely and profoundly developmentally disabled.' *Occupational Therapy Journal of Research*, **1**, 147–160.

—— Bundy, A., Short, M.A. (1983) 'The development and treatment of oral-motor dysfunction: a review of clinical research.' *Physical and Occupational Therapy in Pediatrics*, **3**, 1–13.

Palmer, S., Horn, S. (1978) 'Feeding problems in children.' *In:* Palmer, S., Ekvall, S. (Eds.) *Pediatric Nutrition in Developmental Disorders.* Springfield, IL: Charles C. Thomas, pp. 107–128.

—— Thompson, R.J., Linscheid, T.R. (1975) 'Applied behavior analysis in the treatment of childhood feeding problems.' *Developmental Medicine and Child Neurology*, **17**, 333–339.

Papaila, J.G., Wilmot, D., Grosfeld, J.L., Rescorla, F.J., West, K.W., Vane, D.W. (1989) 'Increased incidence of delayed gastric emptying in children with gastroesophageal reflux. A prospective evaluation.' *Archives of Surgery*, **124**, 933–936.

Patrick, J., Gisel, E. (1990) 'Nutrition for the feeding impaired child.' *Journal of Neurology and Rehabilitation*, **4**, 115–119.

Pearl, R.H., Robie, D.K., Ein, S.H., Shandling, B., Wesson, D.E., Superina, R., Mctaggart, K., Garcia, V.F., O'Connor, J.A., Filler, R.M. (1990) 'Complications of gastroesophageal antireflux surgery in neurologically impaired versus neurologically normal children.' *Journal of Pediatric Surgery*, **25**, 1169–1173.

Pesce, K.A., Wodarski, L.A., Wang, M. (1989) 'Nutritional status of institutionalized children and adolescents with developmental disabilities.' *Research in Developmental Disabilities*, **10**, 33–52.

Reilly, S., Skuse, D. (1992) 'Characteristics and management of feeding problems of young children with cerebral palsy.' *Developmental Medicine and Child Neurology*, **34**, 379–388.

Reyes, A.L., Cash, A.J., Green, S.H., Booth, I.W. (1993) 'Gastrooesophageal reflux in children with cerebral palsy.' *Child: Care, Health and Development*, **19**, 109–118.

Reynell, J. (1979) *Reynell–Zinkin Developmental Scales for Visually Handicapped Children. Part I. Mental Development.* Windsor, Berkshire: NFER.

Riordan, M.M., Iwata, B.A., Finney, J.W., Wohl, M.K., Stanley, A.E. (1984) 'Behavioral assessment and treatment of chronic food refusal in handicapped children.' *Journal of Applied Behavior Analysis*, **17**, 327–341.

Rogers, B.T., Arvedson, J., Msall, M., Demerath, R.R. (1993) 'Hypoxemia during oral feeding of children with severe cerebral palsy.' *Developmental Medicine and Child Neurology*, **35**, 3–10.

Rutter, M., Graham, P., Yule, W. (1970) *A Neuropsychiatric Study in Childhood. Clinics in Developmental Medicine No. 35/36.* London: Spastics International Medical Publications.

Schärli, A.F. (1985) 'Gastroesophageal reflux and severe mental retardation.' *Progress in Pediatric Surgery*, **18**, 84–90.

Smith, C.D., Othersen, H.B., Gogan, N.J., Walker, J.D. (1992) 'Nissen fundoplication in children with profound neurologic disability. High risks and unmet goals.' *Annals of Surgery*, **215**, 654–658.

Sondheimer, J.M., Morris, B.A. (1979) 'Gastroesophageal reflux among severely retarded children.' *Journal of Pediatrics*, **94**, 710–714.

Sonksen, P.M. (1993) 'Effect of severe visual impairment on development.' *In:* Fielder, A.R., Best A.B., Bax M.C.O. (Eds.) *The Management of Visual Impairment in Childhood. Clinics in Developmental Medicine No. 128.* London: Mac Keith Press, pp. 78–90.

31

Stolovitz, P., Gisel, E.G. (1991) 'Circumoral movements in response to three different food textures in children 6 months to 2 years of age.' *Dysphagia*, **6**, 17–25.

Sutphen, J.L., Dillard, V.L. (1992) 'Medium chain triglyceride in the therapy of gastroesophageal reflux.' *Journal of Pediatric Gastroenterology and Nutrition*, **14**, 38–40.

Thommessen, M., Kase, B.F., Riis, G., Heiberg, A. (1991) 'The impact of feeding problems on growth and energy intake in children with cerebral palsy.' *European Journal of Clinical Nutrition*, **45**, 479–487.

Tolia, V., Lin, C-H., Kuhns, L.R. (1992) 'Gastric emptying using three different formulas in infants with gastroesophageal reflux.' *Journal of Pediatric Gastroenterology and Nutrition*, **15**, 297–301.

Tolman, K.G., Jubiz, W., Sannella, J.J., Madsen, J.A., Belsey, R.E., Goldsmith, R.S., Freston, J.W. (1975) 'Osteomalacia associated with anticonvulsant drug therapy in mentally retarded children.' *Pediatrics*, **56**, 45–51.

Van Winckel, M., Robberecht, E. (1993) *Journal of Pediatric Surgery*, **28**, 279. *(Letter.)*

Webb, Y. (1980) 'Feeding and nutrition problems of physically and mentally handicapped children in Britain: a report.' *Journal of Human Nutrition*, **34**, 281–285.

4
THE NUTRITIONAL AND NEURO-DEVELOPMENTAL CONSEQUENCES OF FEEDING DIFFICULTIES IN DISABLED CHILDREN

Lewis Rosenbloom and Peter B. Sullivan

Although it is possible that there is some as yet poorly defined central, possibly neuroendo-crinological, factor which contributes to linear growth failure in children with psychomotor retardation, poor growth in such children has more often been ascribed to their underlying cerebral deficit or physical inactivity than to chronic malnutrition. The result of this is that the nutritional needs of disabled children are frequently neglected. Children with mild cerebral palsy who are mobile although generally below average height are not malnourished, whereas very dependent disabled children are short, and have low weight-for-height, loss of subcutaneous fat and wasted muscles. Episodes of infection or surgery in these disabled children inevitably lead to further weight loss and, because it is difficult to increase the energy intake in children with feeding inefficiency, their convalescence is slow. It is this severely affected group of children that has the greatest problem with feeding from a very early stage in life. Nutritional care is often overlooked in these children in infancy at a critical time of brain growth, potentially compounding the effects of their existing disability (*Lancet* 1990, Boyle 1991).

Malnutrition and the developing brain

In the development of the human brain there is a period of rapid growth which starts in the second trimester of gestation and continues well into the second year of life; up to 85 per cent of the total duration of brain growth occurs in the early postnatal period (Stein and Susser 1985). During this critical time the intricate circuitry that distinguishes the human brain is established in a complex process in which elaboration of neuronal elements and proliferation of oligodendrocytes takes place (Tilton and Miller 1993). It is at this time, therefore, that the developing brain is at its most susceptible to noxious environmental influences including malnutrition. If animals are starved early in life, the weight and the content of lipid and nucleic acid in their brains are less than in well-nourished controls. Similar findings have been reported for human infants, in whom undernutrition severely restricts the amount (but not the chemical composition) of myelin formation (Fox *et al.* 1972, Martínez 1982). It is important to note that the effect of undernutrition on the brain probably relates to its duration relative to the total period of brain growth which is largely complete by 3 years of age.

Malnutrition and psychomotor development

The behavioural apathy, listlessness and reduced motor activity observed among severely undernourished children are well known to paediatricians. Moreover, considerable evidence has been collected over many years attesting to the fact that such undernutrition in early infancy, especially if prolonged, is subsequently associated with a reduction in head circumference and with retardation in psychomotor development (Stoch and Smythe 1963, 1976; Cravioto et al. 1966; Ricciuti 1981; Galler et al. 1984; Grantham-McGregor et al. 1991; Husaini et al. 1991).

Infants and children with a history of severe malnutrition have poorer scores on developmental scales, IQ tests and tests of specific intellectual function than comparison groups (Ricciuti 1981). Also, stunted children, without clinical signs of malnutrition, have been shown to perform comparatively poorly on tests of intersensory integration (Cravioto et al. 1966). Stoch et al. (1982) undertook a prospective 20 year follow-up using psychometric testing and computerized tomography of the brain. These authors contrasted the development of 20 children who had been grossly undernourished during infancy with that of a matched control group. Their findings pointed to a clear relationship between infantile undernutrition, reduced head circumference, suboptimal brain growth and impaired brain function.

The effect of high-calorie supplementation on infant development has also been studied (Grantham-McGregor et al. 1991, Husaini et al. 1991), and results suggest that nutritional intervention has beneficial effects on the motor, but not perhaps on the mental, development of infants and young children. Pollitt et al. (1993), however, studied the effect of early supplementary feeding of Guatemalan infants on cognition over two decades and elegantly demonstrated that correcting early malnutrition can have substantial beneficial effects on subsequent cognitive performance. These authors also noted that the relation of nutrition to cognitive performance is moderated both by the time period of nutritional supplementation and by the larger sociodemographic context in which this takes place.

Although the majority of these studies have taken place in deprived environments in developing countries, their findings are, nevertheless, pertinent to a consideration of the nutritional needs of disabled children. In combination with lack of intellectual and social stimulation, malnutrition does appear to depress mental performance. In children in severely deprived environments these deficits in mental performance recover with adequate food and mental stimulation (Stein and Susser 1985). Similarly, children with an existing compromise of brain function should be provided with adequate nutrition to allow them to maximize their potential for neurodevelopmental progress. It is noteworthy that significant developmental progress in previously undernourished children has been reported to accompany improved nutritional status (Sanders et al. 1990).

The adverse effects of undernutrition are not, of course, confined to impairment of central nervous system function. There is hardly any physiological function which is not compromised by poor nutrition. Although prolonged deficiency of nutrient intake will result in serious malnutrition, it is unclear at what point a reduction in nutrient intake will lead to impairment of vital organ function. Functional impairment may possibly occur at a subclinical level and precede a measurable alteration in body composition.

Malnutrition and the skeletal muscles

Significant changes in skeletal muscle function have been observed in patients with clinically apparent malnutrition (Lopes *et al.* 1982). Nutritional deprivation produces a selective atrophy of type II muscle fibres. This results in a greater proportion of type I fibres, which contract more slowly, tetanize at a lower stimulation frequency and relax more slowly. Moreover, it has been shown that refeeding results in a rapid normalization of muscle function parameters (Russell *et al.* 1983). The effects of such nutrition-induced muscular dysfunction could exacerbate the existing muscular dysfunction in a child with spastic cerebral palsy, but probably of greater significance is the effect on respiratory muscle function. Poorly nourished subjects have lower respiratory muscle strength, abnormal contractility and increased fatiguability of the accessory muscles of respiration. These abnormalities can be reversed over a three month period of nutritional rehabilitation and, in adult patients with chronic obstructive pulmonary disease, this has been shown to be associated with reduced breathlessness (Efthimiou *et al.* 1988). Although no formal studies of muscle function in malnourished children with cerebral palsy have been reported, such impairment of respiratory muscle function would be clearly disadvantageous. Oral-motor dysfunction and gastro-oesophageal reflux combine to render these children susceptible to aspiration and recurrent chest infections, a situation that is exacerbated by an ineffective cough reflex and weak respiratory muscles. Deficient muscle bulk in children with cerebral palsy may predispose to fracture of long bones. Lingam and Joester (1994) reported five children and adolescents with cerebral palsy who developed spontaneous fractures of long bones. They considered that these were due to deficient muscle bulk to the long bones and stresses on these bones imposed by contractures. Shaw *et al.* (1994) have demonstrated that osteopenia in immobile children with cerebral palsy is common and treatable with biphosphonates.

Malnutrition and the immune system

The immunosuppressive effects of malnutrition are also well documented (Chandra 1972, 1983), as are observations that infection is of greater severity, lasts longer and recurs more frequently in malnourished children (Chandra 1979). The severity of nutrition-related dysfunction in the organs of the body depends in part on the rate of cellular proliferation and on protein synthesis in the tissue, and thus the lymphoid system is particularly vulnerable. It is therefore not surprising that undernutrition has profound adverse effects on mucosal and systemic immunity. The most consistent changes in immunocompetence in malnutrition are in cell-mediated immunity. Disturbances in the immune system secondary to malnutrition predispose children with cerebral palsy to infection, particularly of the lungs and the urinary tract. Furthermore, healing of pressure sores is delayed in children with malnutrition. This may be due in part to immunocompromise but also to the circulatory insufficiency typical of undernourished immobile children with cerebral palsy.

Malnutrition and the cardiovascular system

Prolonged circulation time and low cardiac output are known concomitants of malnutrition (Ansari 1987) and, together with poor oxygenation of the blood, are the cause of the pale, cold and mottled extremities so often seen in disabled children. Patrick *et al.* (1986) noted that these changes were corrected by improvement in the nutritional status of the disabled children under their care. These authors also reported that the 10–46 per cent increase in body weight that they achieved in their patients with approximately a 50 per cent increase in energy intake was associated with healing of persistent pressure sores, a fact greatly welcomed by the parents and caretakers of these children.

The nature of malnutrition in disabled children

Energy deficit

On the basis of their experience in the nutritional problems of feeding-impaired disabled children, Patrick and Gisel (1990) emphasize that such problems are, in their opinion, caused primarily by energy deficits rather than by deficits of protein, vitamins or minerals. They affirm that it is because the diet given to disabled children is qualitatively good but deficient in volume that the malnutrition found in such children is rarely associated with either skin changes or hair or mucosal changes. This is, of course, quite different from the clinical picture of childhood malnutrition seen in the developing world where micronutrient deficiencies (such as vitamin A and zinc) together with protein deficiency are much more prominent. The qualitative 'adequacy' but quantitative deficiency of the diets provided for disabled children may also be one of the reasons that such individuals can survive in a moderately malnourished state for many years.

Micronutrient deficiency

Despite the above comments, micronutrient deficiencies, including those of calcium, iron, zinc, vitamin C, vitamin A, riboflavin and thiamin, have been reported in children with developmental disability and may be under-recognized (Phelps 1951, Berg 1973, Garty et al. 1989, Patrick and Gisel 1990, American Dietetic Association 1992). For instance, children with psychomotor retardation may be at a higher risk of subclinical vitamin C deficiency or overt scurvy (Front et al. 1978, Garty et al. 1989).

Garty and colleagues (1989) in Israel reported 12 children with psychomotor retardation (mean age 4.4 years; range 1–10 years) and scurvy. The main presenting clinical features found in these children were either non-specific (irritability, anorexia, weight loss or fever) or involved the limbs ('arthritis', 'osteomyelitis' and tenderness of limbs) and gingivae (swelling and bleeding). The majority of these patients were cared for at home and maintained on a diet consisting of cow's milk and cereals but without fruit and vegetables. The existence of scurvy in these disabled children was not suspected by the referring physicians (hence the initial diagnoses of osteomyelitis and arthritis) and was only made when specifically sought on laboratory investigation. Other laboratory investigations in these children revealed anaemia, folic acid deficiency, iron deficiency and nutritional rickets. Awareness of this easily treatable, and possibly under-recognized condition is necessary among those caring for the nutritional needs of disabled children. It is noteworthy in this context that low plasma vitamin C concentration per se is not diagnostic of scurvy and can be related to a temporary deficiency of vitamin C or increased utilization. However, the lack of urinary excretion of vitamin C after an ascorbic acid load does indicate depletion of vitamin C and not just low intake.

Iron deficiency

Of all the micronutrients influencing neurodevelopmental status, the deficiency of iron is perhaps the one which has been studied most. Walter *et al.* (1989) showed that, on psycho-motor testing, items which relate to balance in the standing position and walking were ac-complished by significantly fewer infants with anaemia than controls. The drawback of this study from Chile was a follow-up period of only two to three months. Thus, it is difficult to determine whether adverse effects of iron deficiency anaemia persist beyond infancy. Walter (1993), therefore, assessed a group of children who were iron deficient at 12 months of age and tested them again at 5–6 years of age. The battery of tests used encompassed a general intelligence test (the Stanford–Binet), a test of fine and gross motor performance (the Bruininks–Oseretsky test of motor proficiency), a test of psycholinguistic capabilities (Illinois), a test of visual-motor integration (Beery), and an educational school preparedness scale (Woodcock–Johnson preschool scale). At follow-up the formerly anaemic children showed a persistence of lower performances when compared with their iron-replete peers. Aukett *et al.* (1986) undertook a double-blind randomized intervention study to determine the effect of oral iron treatment on psychomotor development in anaemic children living in an inner-city, underprivileged environment. While these authors found that treatment with iron increased both weight gain and psychomotor development, they recognized that it is unlikely that iron deficiency was the only factor in the slower development of children in an underprivileged environment. It is, however, a factor that can be easily identified and treated. There is now sufficient evidence that iron deficiency is detrimental to neurodevelop-mental progress and that if left untreated, deficiencies will persist; an iron-deficient state at the time of rapid brain growth does appear to impair brain function, and such effects may remain (Palti *et al.* 1985). Conversely, treatment of iron deficiency can produce a rapid im-provement in developmental scores in infants (Oski *et al.* 1983). Recently, Idjradinata and Pollitt (1993) showed that although iron-deficient anaemic infants perform worse in tests of motor and mental development than do iron-sufficient infants of a comparable age, such developmental delay can be reversed in iron-deficient infants by treatment with ferrous sulphate.

Disabled children may be at greater risk of iron deficiency as their diet is often limited, and especially so if the diet is based largely on cow's milk. Iron deficiency anaemia is well described in infants fed predominantly on cow's milk and is related to the poor concentration and bioavailability of iron in cow's milk (Sadowitz and Oski 1983, Penrod *et al.* 1990, Pizarro *et al.* 1991, American Academy of Pediatrics 1992). Tunnessen and Oski (1987) found that 22.2 per cent of infants fed whole cow's milk after 6 months of age had evidence of iron insufficiency (lower mean corpuscular volume, lower ferritin levels and higher free erythro-cyte protoporphyrin levels) at 12 months of age. They concluded that the results of their study of infants between 6 and 12 months of age indicated that low iron content of whole cow's milk was the primary factor responsible for iron inadequacy in their patients.

REFERENCES

American Academy of Pediatrics Committee on Nutrition (1992) 'The use of whole cow's milk in infancy.' *Pediatrics*, **89**, 1105–1109.

American Dietetic Association (1992) 'Position of the American Dietetic Association: nutrition in comprehensive program planning for persons with developmental disabilities.' *Journal of the American Dietetic Association*, **92**, 613–615.

Ansari, A. (1987) 'Syndromes of cardiac cachexia and the cachectic heart.' *Progress in Cardiovascular Disease*, **30**, 45–60.

Aukett, M.A., Parks, Y.A., Scott, P.H., Wharton, B.A. (1986) 'Treatment with iron increases weight gain and psychomotor development.' *Archives of Disease in Childhood*, **61**, 849–857.

Berg, K. (1973) 'Nutrition of children with reduced physical activity due to cerebral palsy.' *Bibliotheca 'Nutritio et Dieta'*, No. 19, 12–20.

Boyle, J.T. (1991) 'Nutritional management of the developmentally disabled child.' *Pediatric Surgery International*, **6**, 76–81.

Chandra, R.K. (1972) 'Immunocompetence in undernutrition.' *Journal of Pediatrics*, **81**, 1194–1200.

—— (1979) 'Nutritional deficiency and susceptibility to infection.' *Bulletin of the World Health Organization*, **57**, 167–177.

—— (1983) 'Nutrition, immunity, and infection: present knowledge and future directions.' *Lancet*, **1**, 688–691.

Cravioto, J., DeLicardie, E.R., Birch, H.G. (1966) 'Nutrition, growth and neurointegrative development: an experimental and ecologic study.' *Pediatrics*, **38** (Suppl. 2, Pt. 2), 319–372.

Efthimiou, J., Fleming, J., Gomes, C., Spiro, S.G. (1988) 'The effect of supplementary oral nutrition in poorly nourished patients with chronic obstructive pulmonary disease.' *American Review of Respiratory Disease*, **137**, 1075–1082.

Fox, J.H., Fishman, M.A., Dodge, P.R., Prensky, A.L. (1972) 'The effect of malnutrition on human central nervous system myelin.' *Neurology*, **22**, 1213–1216.

Front, D., Hardoff, R., Levy, J., Benderly, A. (1978) 'Bone scintigraphy in scurvy.' *Journal of Nuclear Medicine*, **19**, 916–917.

Galler, J.R., Ramsey, F., Solimano, G. (1984) 'The influence of early malnutrition on subsequent behavioral development. III. Learning disabilities as a sequel to malnutrition.' *Pediatric Research*, **18**, 309–313.

Garty, B.Z., Danon, Y.L., Grunebaum, M., Nitzan, M. (1989) 'Scurvy in children with severe psychomotor retardation.' *International Pediatrics*, **4**, 279–282.

Grantham-McGregor, S.M., Powell, C.A., Walker, S.P., Himes, J.H. (1991) 'Nutritional supplementation, psychosocial stimulation, and mental development of stunted children: the Jamaican Study.' *Lancet*, **338**, 1–5.

Husaini, M.A., Karyadi, L., Husaini, Y.K., Sandjaja, Karyadi, D., Pollitt, E. (1991) 'Developmental effects of short-term suplementary feeding in nutritionally-at-risk Indonesian infants.' *American Journal of Clinical Nutrition*, **54**, 799–804.

Idjradinata, P., Pollitt, E. (1993) 'Reversal of developmental delays in iron-deficient anaemic infants treated with iron.' *Lancet*, **341**, 1–4.

Lancet (1990) 'Growth and nutrition in children with cerebral palsy.' *Lancet*, **335**, 1253–1254.

Lingam, S., Joester, J. (1994) 'Spontaneous fractures in children and adolescents with cerebral palsy.' *British Medical Journal*, **309**, 265.

Lopes, J., Russell, D.McR., Whitwell, J., Jeejeebhoy, K.N. (1982) 'Skeletal muscle function in malnutrition.' *American Journal of Clinical Nutrition*, **36**, 602–610.

Martínez, M. (1982) 'Myelin lipids in the developing cerebrum, cerebellum, and brain stem of normal and undernourished children.' *Journal of Neurochemistry*, **39**, 1684–1692.

Oski, F.A., Honig, A.S., Helu, B., Howanitz, P. (1983) 'Effect of iron therapy on behavior performance in nonanemic, iron-deficient infants.' *Pediatrics*, **71**, 877–880.

Palti, H., Meijer, A., Adler, B. (1985) 'Learning achievement and behavior at school of anemic and non-anemic infants.' *Early Human Development*, **10**, 217–223.

Patrick, J., Gisel, E. (1990) 'Nutrition for the feeding impaired child.' *Journal of Neurology and Rehabilitation*, **4**, 115–119.

—— Boland, M., Stoski, D., Murray, G.E. (1986) 'Rapid correction of wasting in children with cerebral palsy.' *Developmental Medicine and Child Neurology*, **28**, 734–739.

Penrod, J.C., Anderson, K., Acosta, P.B. (1990) 'Impact on iron status of introducing cow's milk in the second six months of life.' *Journal of Pediatric Gastroenterology and Nutrition*, **10**, 462–467.

Phelps, W.M. (1951) 'Dietary requirements in cerebral palsy.' *Journal of the American Dietetic Association*, **27**, 869–870.

Pizarro, F., Yip, R., Dallman, P.R., Olivares, M., Hertrampf, E., Walter, T. (1991) 'Iron status with different

38

infant feeding regimens: relevance to screening and prevention of iron deficiency.' *Journal of Pediatrics*, **118**, 687–692.

Pollitt, E., Gorman, K.S., Engle, P.L., Martorell, R., Rivera, J. (1993) *Early Supplementary Feeding and Cognition: Effects Over Two Decades. Monographs of the Society for Research in Child Development, Vol. 58, No.7. (Serial No. 235.)*

Ricciuti, H. (1981) 'Developmental consequences of malnutrition in early childhood.' *In:* Lewis, M., Rosenblum, N. (Eds.) *The Uncommon Child: the Genesis of Behavior.* New York: Plenum.

Russell, D.McR., Leiter, L.A., Whitwell, J., Marliss, E.B., Jeejeebhoy, K.N. (1983) 'Skeletal muscle function during hypocaloric diets and fasting: a comparison with standard nutritional assessment parameters.' *American Journal of Clinical Nutrition*, **37**, 133–138.

Sadowitz, P.D., Oski, F.A. (1983) 'Iron status and infant feeding practices in an urban ambulatory center.' *Pediatrics*, **72**, 33–36.

Sanders, K.D., Cox, K., Cannon, R., Blanchard, D., Pitcher, J., Papathakis, P., Varella, L., Maughan, R. (1990) 'Growth response to enteral feeding by children with cerebral palsy.' *Journal of Parenteral and Enteral Nutrition*, **14**, 23–26.

Shaw, N.J., White, C.P., Fraser, W.D., Rosenbloom, L. (1994) 'Osteopenia in cerebral palsy.' *Archives of Disease in Childhood*, **71**, 235–238.

Stein, Z., Susser, M. (1985) 'Effects of early nutrition on neurological and mental competence in human beings.' *Psychological Medicine*, **15**, 717–726.

Stoch, M.B.,Smythe, P.M. (1963) 'Does undernutrition during infancy inhibit brain growth and subsequent intellectual development?' *Archives of Disease in Childhood*, **38**, 546–552.

——— ——— (1976) '15-year developmental study on effects of severe undernutrition during infancy on subsequent physical growth and intellectual functioning.' *Archives of Disease in Childhood*, **51**, 327–336.

——— ——— Moodie, A.D.,Bradshaw, D. (1982) 'Psychosocial outcome and CT findings after gross undernourishment during infancy: a 20-year developmental study.' *Developmental Medicine and Child Neurology*, **24**, 419–436.

Tilton, A.C., Miller, M.D. (1993) 'Nutritional support of the developmentally disabled child.' *In:* Suskind, R.M., Lewinter-Suskind, L. (Eds.) *Textbook of Pediatric Nutrition.* New York: Raven Press, pp. 485–491.

Tunnessen, W.W., Oski, F.A. (1987) 'Consequences of starting whole cow milk at 6 months of age.' *Journal of Pediatrics*, **111**, 813–816.

Walter, T., (1993) 'Impact of iron deficiency on cognition in infancy and childhood.' *European Journal of Clinical Nutrition*, **47**, 307–316.

——— de Andraca, I., Chadud, P., Perales, C.G. (1989) 'Iron deficiency anemia: adverse effects on infant psychomotor development.' *Pediatrics*, **84**, 7–17.

5
THE RESPIRATORY CONSEQUENCES OF NEUROLOGICAL DEFICIT

Ben (N.J.) Shaw

Children who have neurological damage, in particular cerebral palsy, may have disordered feeding and swallowing patterns which predispose them to the development of recurrent respiratory disease (Logemann 1986, Loughlin 1989, Phelan 1990). In patients who are institutionalized because of severe mental retardation (many of whom have cerebral palsy), up to 46 per cent of deaths are associated with lower respiratory tract infection, and up to 15 per cent of sudden deaths are associated with non-epileptic asphyxia (Carter and Jancar 1983).

A number of factors may make the child with neuromotor impairment liable to respiratory difficulties. If the impairment severely restricts mobility, if the respiratory musculature is weak, if the ability to cough is diminished, and/or if obesity is present, tidal volume may be reduced and respiratory failure ensue. Kyphoscoliosis causing chest wall deformity can result in reduced lung volume. A child with cerebral palsy born very preterm may have coexisting bronchopulmonary dysplasia, which is associated with an increased risk of symptoms of obstructive airway disease in later life. As with any child, a family history of atopy increases the risk of asthma, while parental smoking (particularly maternal, both ante- and postnatally) has been shown to increase the risk of respiratory symptoms in the first 2–3 years of life (Milner 1993).

The effects of malnutrition on respiratory status that have been described in adults are also likely to occur in the motor impaired child who is malnourished, possibly as a result of poor feeding. The respiratory muscles are subject to the same catabolic changes as other skeletal muscles during starvation. In studies of adults with a severe reduction in body weight, atrophy and weakness of the diaphragm have been reported (Arora and Rochester 1982), and in protein depleted patients there is significant impairment of respiratory muscle strength, reduced vital capacity and reduced peak flow rate (Hill 1988). Further studies in adults have shown that starvation results in a reduced ventilatory response to hypoxia and reduced inspiratory flow (Doekel *et al.* 1976, Weissman *et al.* 1983), and that malnutrition is associated with increased bacterial colonization of the airways and their impaired resistance to infection (Niederman *et al.* 1984). Protein calorie malnutrition results in impaired cell mediated immunity, reduced immunoglobulin turnover and a reduction in secretory IgA (Stiehm 1980, Peck and Alexander 1990). In experimental animals subjected to malnutrition there is a reduction in alveolar phagocyte function and a reduction in clearance of various micro-organisms from the airways (Shennib *et al.* 1984).

Parenteral administration of specific nutrients may exacerbate respiratory difficulties.

Carbohydrate administration increases carbon dioxide production, which in the absence of a compensatory increase in ventilation may result in carbon dioxide retention and possibly respiratory failure (Rodriguez *et al.* 1985). Parenterally administered fat emulsions have been associated with increased respiratory morbidity in preterm infants, although their effect in children with neurodevelopmental disorders is unknown (Pereira *et al.* 1980). Amino acid infusions may result in increased minute volume and ventilatory drive which may increase respiratory distress if the patient's lung function is borderline normal (Weissman *et al.* 1983). Specific nutrient deficiencies may also contribute to respiratory morbidity. Phosphate deficiency may result in reduced diaphragmatic function (Aubier *et al.* 1985) and magnesium deficiency may result in reduced respiratory muscle strength (Benotti and Bistrian 1989).

Swallowing and feeding

Oral feeding depends on the coordination of the child's swallowing and breathing (see Chapter 2). Under normal circumstances the pharynx is completely emptied of food and saliva by the process of swallowing, and the cough reflex exists to ensure that if any food does remain it does not enter the larynx. Tongue action is vital in the initiation of the swallowing reflex, so if tongue coordination is poor, the reflex may not occur at the correct time and aspiration may result.

In cerebral palsy the rhythm of swallowing can be absent because damage to the brainstem and cranial nerve nuclei leads to neuromuscular incoordination and paralysis. There is overfilling of the mouth and pharynx with food spilling in to the larynx, saliva accumulates, and drooling and gurgling breathing occur. If the nasopharynx is not closed during swallowing, nasal flooding can occur and liquids escape from the nostrils (Ardran *et al.* 1965). The cough reflex may be depressed due to repeated stimulation of receptors in the larynx and trachea. Gastro-oesophageal reflux and a nasogastric tube *in situ* serve to worsen the situation. Hypersensitivity of vagally mediated irritant receptors have been reported to produce apnoea and bradycardia in the dog (Angell-James and de Burgh Daly 1973) and in the human child (Perkett and Vaughan 1982).

Respiratory symptoms during oral feeding

Young infants with neuromotor impairment, especially those born preterm, may present with apnoea and bradycardia during oral feeding, whereas older children may cough or choke (Loughlin 1989). Apnoea and bradycardia occurring some time after feeds can be secondary to gastro-oesophageal reflux. The apnoea is probably vagally mediated and may either be central or obstructive. It is a protective mechanism but if prolonged will produce hypoxia and bradycardia. Vagally mediated apnoea may also occur if milk feeds trickle into the nasopharynx (Plaxico and Loughlin 1981). In infants born preterm a raised arterial carbon dioxide concentration may result in increased respiratory drive which may impair sucking and swallowing, and infants with bronchopulmonary dysplasia may become cyanosed when feeding (Garg *et al.* 1988, Timms *et al.* 1993).

In the older child, symptoms include chronic recurrent cough, congestion and wheeze, all of which may be exacerbated by feeding (Fisher *et al.* 1981). Children who have extensor dystonia may have upper airway narrowing, resulting in respiratory distress and stridor with feeding (Couriel *et al.* 1993). Hypotonia can result in the tongue and jaw falling backwards causing upper airway obstruction and stridor (Couriel *et al.* 1993). Auscultation of the pharynx and trachea during swallowing and of the lungs before and after swallowing may reveal rattling and gurgling due to retained food in the nasopharynx or aspirated food.

Aspiration
Children with an impaired swallow have a poorly protected airway and are at high risk of aspiration which is defined as entry of material into the airway below the true vocal cords (Logemann 1986). Aspiration can occur before, during or after the swallow (Logemann 1985). Aspiration before the swallow may be due to poor tongue control or delay in or absence of the triggering of the swallow reflex. If there is poor tongue control during the oral preparation of food and oral stage of swallowing when the airway is still open, the food bolus rolls back into the pharynx and directly into the airway. The clinical effect of this will depend on the posture of the child when feeding and on the amount and consistency of food presented to the child. If the swallowing reflex is impaired, the larynx remains open for too long despite food entering the oropharynx, resulting in possible aspiration.

Aspiration during the swallow is a result of *reduced* laryngeal closure rather than delayed closure, the former often being a result of vocal cord paralysis.

Aspiration after the swallow can have a variety of causes. Food remaining in the pharynx as a result of inefficient swallowing can enter the airway. Rare anatomical abnormalities such as oesophageal fistulae or diverticulae may also result in residual food or liquids entering the airway. Finally, gastro-oesophageal reflux occurring immediately or some time after the meal may result in aspiration after the swallow.

Aspiration causes hypoxaemia (Rogers *et al.* 1993), closure of the distal airways (Colebatch and Halmagyi 1962, Schwartz *et al.* 1980), reduction of lung compliance, and ventilation perfusion mismatch (Lewis *et al.* 1971, Conn and Barker 1984). Pneumonitis can result, although reflex hypoxaemia may occur in its absence (Schwartz *et al.* 1980).

The pathological findings of aspiration depend on the type and amount of food aspirated. Inhaled milk produces an acute inflammatory reaction in the airways and alveoli with neutrophil and macrophage infiltration. Macrophages become foamy and vacuolated as they are filled with fat (Phelan 1990). Eventually a granulomatous reaction followed by fibrosis may occur. Aspiration of gastric contents may cause more inflammation due to the lower pH of material entering the airway than is the case with swallowed food (Mendelson 1946).

The respiratory symptoms and signs of aspiration depend on the amount of food aspirated and whether it is recurrent. Cough, rattly breathing, wheeze and tachypnoea may occur. On examination of the chest, wheeze and crackles may be heard posteriorly and the chest may be hyperinflated (Loughlin 1989, Phelan 1990). Symptoms may occur during or after feeds; however, lung damage is possible without symptoms if there is an impaired cough reflex (Phelan 1990). Wheezing may be the main symptom of gastro-oesophageal reflux and may occur as a result of vagal reflexes rather than as a result of the gastric contents actually entering the airway (Mansfield and Stein 1978, Euler *et al.* 1979, Berquist *et al.* 1981*a*, Loughlin 1989, Phelan 1990). As mentioned above, life threatening apnoea and bradycardia may occur. With severe inhalation, secondary infection and pneumonia supervene giving rise to fever, cough, malaise, tachypnoea and sometimes cyanosis (Taniguchi and Moyer 1994).

Recurrent aspiration produces intercurrent wheeze and cough. When recurrent aspiration occurs, respiratory symptoms and signs may be a result of secondary infection rather than the acute event (Loughlin 1989, Phelan 1990). Eventually chronic interstitial pneumonitis and fibrosis may develop which results in persistent cough, recurrent fever, malaise, shortness of breath, tachypnoea and failure to thrive (Phelan 1990). Stridor produced by tracheomalacia secondary to tracheal injury can occur (Loughlin 1989).

In the most severe cases persistent atelectasis, bronchiectasis with a chronic productive cough or bronchiolitis obliterans may follow (Loughlin 1989, Phelan 1990).

The radiological consequences of aspiration depend on the age of the child, the duration and severity of inhalation, and the presence of secondary infection. Gravity determines the distribution of the radiographic lesions. On the chest radiograph hilar shadowing and hyperinflation can often be seen with patchy or uniform opacification in the lung fields. If the child is usually fed lying down, posterior upper and lower lobes, particularly on the right, tend to be affected. If the child is mobile, both lower lobes, lingula and right middle lobe are most often involved.

Gastro-oesophageal reflux can occur in up to 75 per cent of children with cerebral palsy, sometimes in the absence of vomiting (Booth 1992). Recurrent aspiration or the presence of coexisting lung disease such as bronchopulmonary dysplasia or asthma may cause chest hyperinflation which alters the relationship between the diaphragm and the lower oesophageal sphincter and may increase reflux. Xanthines such as theophylline may lower the tone of the lower oesophageal sphincter and should be used with caution in children with neuromotor impairment (Berquist *et al.* 1981*b*).

Assessment

Assessment of the neuromotor impaired child for respiratory sequelae involves taking an appropriate history, examining the patient, and where appropriate performing special investigations. In the history, important points include the child's feeding pattern, and whether she chokes or vomits. The nature, frequency and severity of respiratory symptoms together with any trigger factors for these symptoms should be determined. Enquiry should also be made about the number of previous hospital admissions, current medications, perinatal course and family history of atopy and smoking. The child's weight and length should be measured, any chest or spinal deformity should be noted, and the pattern of breathing and presence of cough should be observed.

A chest radiograph is mandatory. Computerized tomography of the chest may provide further information in the presence of severe symptoms such as productive cough where there are only minor or no obvious abnormalities on the plain chest radiograph. Aspiration may be identified by a modified barium swallow keeping the oral cavity in view during the procedure (Logemann 1986). The control of food in the oropharynx, bolus production and proportion swallowed can be observed. The state of the cough reflex and presence of gastro-oesophageal reflux can be determined (Kramer 1989; Dodds *et al.* 1990*a,b*). Isotope milk scanning is not a particularly sensitive method for detecting aspiration (McVeagh *et al.* 1987). If reflux is suspected, lower oesophageal pH monitoring can be undertaken. Bronchoscopy can be performed to obtain secretions which can be examined for fat-laden macrophages which may indicate reflux (Mendelson 1946). Bronchoscopy will also yield information with regard to vocal cord function and the presence of anatomical abnormalities, and can be used therapeutically to clear the airway.

Pulse oximetry has been performed in children with food refusal or cough and fatigue during feeding (Rogers *et al.* 1993). Resting oxygen saturation may be related to the type and texture of food being taken. Pulse oximetry can be used to assess different feeding regimes and may provide information which may help to decide if gastrostomy tube feeds are indicated (Rogers *et al.* 1993).

Intermittent hypoxia is not only important as an indicator of aspiration during feeding but also may predispose to poor nutritional status, developmental delay, cognitive defects and right heart failure. Improved oxygenation may make the child more alert and active (Rogers *et al.* 1993).

Treatment

An attempt should be made to treat the causes of respiratory problems in the neuro-logically impaired child. A speech therapist may diagnose a physical problem or the reason for aspiration and may establish safe swallowing by giving advice regarding posture when feeding and the consistency of food to use. Various exercises can be introduced in the older child to stimulate the swallowing reflex, produce laryngeal adduction during swallowing and clear food debris from the larynx and pharynx after swallowing (Logemann 1986).

Nasogastric feeding or gastrostomy feeding may be instituted to bypass the pharynx. Antireflux medication such as feed thickeners or Gaviscon together with prokinetic agents can be tried for gastro-oesophageal reflux, and in severe cases fundoplication may have to be performed (Spitz *et al.* 1993).

The respiratory *consequences* in the neuromotor impaired child should also be treated. Physiotherapy may help the child with chronic suppurative lung disease. Continuous low dose antibiotic therapy may prevent recurrent respiratory infections. Episodes of wheeze may respond to bronchodilators administered via a delivery system appropriate for the capability of the child (for example a spacer device and mask). If there is concurrent asthma, or if wheeze is the predominant feature, courses of oral steroids and possibly prophylactic inhaled steroids may suppress respiratory symptoms.

Conclusion

In the child with neurological deficit, many factors may predispose to the development of respiratory sequelae. Respiratory assessment is essential to determine if there is any significant respiratory disease, what the cause(s) of this may be and what treatment, if any, is required. It has been suggested that feeding problems in children with neurodevelopmental disability should be dealt with by a multidisciplinary team which should involve a clinician with an interest in respiratory paediatrics in order that respiratory disease can be detected and treated promptly in these patients (Couriel *et al.* 1993).

REFERENCES

Angell-James, J.E., de Burgh Daly, M. (1973) 'The interaction of reflexes elicited by stimulation of carotid body chemoreceptors and receptors in the nasal mucosa affecting respiration and pulse interval in the dog.' *Journal of Physiology*, **229**, 133–149.

Ardran, G.M., Benson, P.F., Butler, N.R., Ellis, H.L., McKendrick, T. (1965) 'Congenital dysphagia resulting from dysfunction of the pharyngeal musculature. A clinical and radiological study.' *Developmental Medicine and Child Neurology*, **7**, 157–166.

Arora, N.S., Rochester, D.F. (1982) 'Effects of body weight and muscularity on human diaphragm muscle mass, thickness, and area.' *Journal of Applied Physiology*, **52**, 64–70.

Aubier, M., Murciano, D., Lecocguic, Y., Viires, N., Jacquens, Y., Squara, P., Pariente, R. (1985) 'Effect of hypophosphatemia on the diaphragmatic contractility in patients with acute respiratory failure.' *New England Journal of Medicine*, **313**, 420–424.

Benotti, P.N., Bistrian, B. (1989) 'Metabolic and nutritional aspects of weaning from mechanical ventilation.' *Critical Care Medicine*, **17**, 181–185.

Berquist, W.E., Rachelefsky, G.S., Kadden, M., Siegel, S.C., Katz, R.M., Fonkalsrud, E.W., Ament, M.E. (1981*a*) 'Gastroesophageal reflux-associated recurrent pneumonia and chronic asthma in children.' *Pediatrics*, **68**, 29–35.

—— —— —— —— Mickey, M.R., Ament, M.E. (1981*b*) 'Effect of theophylline on gastroesophageal reflux in normal adults.' *Journal of Allergy and Clinical Immunology*, **67**, 407–411.

Booth, I.W. (1992) 'Silent gastro-oesophageal reflux: how much do we miss?' *Archives of Disease in Childhood*, **67**, 1325–1327. *(Annotation.)*

Carter, G., Jancar, J. (1983) 'Mortality in the mentally handicapped: a 50 year survey at the Stoke Park Group of Hospitals (1930–1980).' *Journal of Mental Deficiency Research*, **27**, 143–156.

Colebatch, H.J.H., Halmagyi, D.F.J. (1962) 'Reflex airway reaction to fluid aspiration.' *Journal of Applied Physiology*, **17**, 787–794.

Conn, A.W., Barker, G.A. (1984) 'Fresh water drowning and near-drowning—an update.' *Canadian Anaesthetists' Society Journal*, **31**, S38–S44.

Couriel, J.M., Bisset, R., Miller, R., Thomas, A., Clarke, M. (1993) 'Assessment of feeding problems in neurodevelopmental handicap: a team approach.' *Archives of Disease in Childhood*, **69**, 609–613.

Dodds, W.J., Logemann, J.A., Stewart, E.T. (1990*a*) 'Radiological assessment of abnormal oral and pharyngeal phases of swallowing.' *American Journal of Roentgenology*, **154**, 965–974.

—— Stewart, E.T., Logemann, J.A. (1990*b*) 'Physiology and radiology of the normal oral and pharyngeal phases of swallowing.' *American Journal of Roentgenology*, **154**, 953–963.

Doekel, R.C. Jr., Zwillich, C.W., Scoggin, C.H., Kryger, M., Weil, J.V. (1976) 'Clinical semi-starvation. Depression of hypoxic ventilatory response.' *New England Journal of Medicine*, **295**, 358–361.

Euler, A.R., Byrne, W.J., Ament, M.E., Fonkalsrud, E.W., Strobel, C.T., Siegel, S.C., Katz, R.M., Rachelefsky, G.S. (1979) 'Recurrent pulmonary disease in children: a complication of gastroesophageal reflux.' *Pediatrics*, **63**, 47–51.

Fisher, S.E., Painter, M., Milmoe, G. (1981) 'Swallowing disorders in infancy.' *Pediatric Clinics of North America*, **28**, 845–853.

Garg, M., Kurzner, S.I., Bautista, D.B., Keens, T.G. (1988) 'Clinically unsuspected hypoxia during sleep and feeding in infants with bronchopulmonary dysplasia.' *Pediatrics*, **81**, 635–642.

Hill, G.L. (1988) 'Body composition research at the University of Auckland—some implications for modern surgical practice.' *Australian and New Zealand Journal of Surgery*, **58**, 13–21.

Kramer, S.S. (1989) 'Radiologic examination of the swallowing impaired child.' *Dysphagia*, **3**, 117–125.

Lewis, R.T., Burgess, J.H., Hampson, L.G. (1971) 'Cardiorespiratory studies in critical illness. Changes in aspiration pneumonitis.' *Archives of Surgery*, **103**, 335–340.

Logemann, J.A. (1985) 'Aspiration in head and neck surgical patients.' *Annals of Otology, Rhinology and Laryngology*, **94**, 373–376.

—— (1986) 'Treatment for aspiration related to dysphagia: an overview.' *Dysphagia*, **1**, 34–38.

Loughlin, G.M. (1989) 'Respiratory consquences of dysfunctional swallowing and aspiration.' *Dysphagia*, **3**, 126–130.

McVeagh, P., Howman-Giles, R., Kemp, A. (1987) 'Pulmonary aspiration studied by radionuclide milk scanning and barium swallow roentgenography.' *American Journal of Diseases of Children*, **141**, 917–921.

Mansfield, L.E., Stein, M.R. (1978) 'Gastroesophageal reflux and asthma: a possible reflex mechanism.' *Annals of Allergy*, **41**, 224–226.

Mendelson, C.L. (1946) 'The aspiration of stomach contents into the lungs during obstetric anesthesia.' *American Journal of Obstetrics and Gynecology*, **52**, 191–204.

Milner, A.D. (1993) 'The respiratory affects of maternal smoking during pregnancy.' *Paediatric Respiratory Medicine*, **1** (4), 16–19.

Niederman, M.S., Merrill, W.W., Ferranti, R.D., Pagano, K.M., Palmer, L.B., Reynolds, H.Y. (1984) 'Nutritional status and bacterial binding in the lower respiratory tract in patients with chronic tracheostomy.' *Annals of Internal Medicine*, **100**, 795–800.

Peck, M.D., Alexander, J.W. (1990) 'The use of immunologic tests to predict outcome in surgical patients.' *Nutrition*, **6**, 16–19.

Pereira, G.R., Fox, W.W., Stanley, C.A., Baker, L., Schwartz, J.G. (1980) 'Decreased oxygenation and hyperlipemia during intravenous fat infusions in premature infants.' *Pediatrics*, **66**, 26–30.

Perkett, E.A., Vaughan, R.L. (1982) 'Evidence for a laryngeal chemoreflex in some human preterm infants.' *Acta Paediatrica Scandanavica*, **71**, 969–972.

Phelan, P.D. (1990) 'Pulmonary complications of inhalation.' *In:* Phelan, P.D., Landau, L.I., Olinsky, A. (Eds.) *Respiratory Illness in Children, 3rd Edn.* Oxford: Blackwell Scientific, pp. 234–249.

Plaxico, D.T., Loughlin, G.M. (1981) 'Nasopharyngeal reflux and neonatal apnea.' *American Journal of Diseases of Children*, **135**, 793–794.

Rodriquez, J.L., Askanazi, J., Weissman, C., Hensle, T.W., Rosenbaum, S.H., Kinney, J.M. (1985) 'Ventilatory and metabolic effects of glucose infusions.' *Chest*, **88**, 512–518.

Rogers, B.T., Arvedson, J., Msall, M., Demerath, R.R. (1993) 'Hypoxemia during oral feeding of children with severe cerebral palsy.' *Developmental Medicine and Child Neurology*, **35**, 3–10.

Schwartz, D.J., Wynne, J.W., Gibbs, C.P., Hood, C.I., Kuck, E.J. (1980) 'The pulmonary consequences of aspiration of gastric contents at pH values greater than 2.5.' *American Review of Respiratory Disease*, **121**, 119–126.

Shennib, H., Chiu, R.C-J., Mulder, D.S., Lough, J.O. (1984) 'Depression and delayed recovery of alveolar macrophage function during starvation and refeeding.' *Surgery, Gynecology and Obstetrics*, **158**, 535–540.

Spitz, L., Roth, K., Kiely, E.M., Brereton, R.J., Drake, D.P., Milla, P.J. (1993) 'Operation for gastro-oesophageal reflux associated with severe mental retardation.' *Archives of Disease in Childhood*, **68**, 347–351.

Stiehm, E.R. (1980) 'Humoral immunity in malnutrition' *Federation Proceedings*, **39**, 3093–3097.

Taniguchi, M.H., Moyer, R.S. (1994) 'Assessment of risk factors for pneumonia in dysphagic children: significance of videofluoroscopic swallowing evaluation.' *Developmental Medicine and Child Neurology*, **36**, 495–502.

Timms, B.J.M., DiFiore, J.M., Martin, R.J., Miller, M.J. (1993) 'Increased respiratory drive as an inhibitor of oral feeding of preterm infants.' *Journal of Pediatrics*, **123**, 127–131.

Weissman, C., Askanazi, J., Rosenbaum, S., Hyman, A.I., Milic-Emili, J., Kinney, J.M. (1983) 'Amino acids and respiration.' Annals of Internal Medicine, 98, 41–44.

6
THE THERAPEUTIC APPROACH TO THE CHILD WITH FEEDING DIFFICULTY: I. ASSESSMENT

Lynn S. Wolf and Robin P. Glass

Children with neurological impairment frequently have significant problems in the areas of growth, nutrition and feeding (Bax 1989, Griggs *et al.* 1989, Reilly and Skuse 1992). The goal of a feeding assessment is to identify the factors underlying these feeding and growth problems, while highlighting the child's strengths. This information then forms the basis of a treatment plan which minimizes the risk for aspiration, optimizes nutrition, and improves the quantity and/or quality of oral intake.

Feeding is clearly a 'multi-system' skill. It requires anatomic integrity, neuromuscular control and coordination, sensory perception, adequate gastro-intestinal function, cardio-respiratory support, and integration from the autonomic nervous system. It is also heavily intertwined with behavioural responses (Wolf and Glass 1992, Glass and Wolf 1993). Therefore, the assessment of feeding necessitates a multidisciplinary approach (Jones 1989, Arvedson and Brodsky 1993, Kramer and Eicher 1993, Tuchman and Walter 1994). While this may be an informal arrangement, many centers are now developing specific feeding teams or feeding clinics to bring multiple specialties together for assessment and management of the often complex feeding problems seen in children with neurologic impairment. If breadth of expertise is not available, the quality of the feeding services offered will be limited.

This chapter will focus on the clinical assessment, or direct observation of feeding, by the 'feeding specialist'. The feeding specialist is generally an occupational therapist or speech therapist, but at times may also be a qualified nurse or physical therapist. Although information gathered through the child's history or interview with caretakers is important to the assessment process, the value of direct observation of feeding is clear (Kramer and Eicher 1993, Lefton-Greif 1994). During a comprehensive evaluation, a skilled therapist can identify abnormal sensory, motor and oral-motor patterns, and assess their impact on the feeding process. The skilled therapist frequently also observes important behavioral or physiologic responses during feeding that suggest the need for further specialized tests or evaluation by the feeding team. For this reason, a clinical feeding assessment in the initial stages of the evaluation may expedite the entire evaluation process.

The type of feeding problems covered in this text cross all pediatric age ranges, though feeding methods and expected skills vary with age. Regardless of the child's age, all feeding concerns identified by the parents or medical staff should be seriously considered and the evaluation process initiated swiftly if problems do not resolve spontaneously. Not only

47

can weight gain and growth quickly become compromised, potentially affecting development, but the frustration and stress of ongoing feeding problems can be overwhelming to families.

Six areas should be addressed during the clinical assessment of feeding: behavior, tactile responses, general motoric control, oral-motor control, swallowing, and the coordination of oral activity with swallowing and breathing. Each of these components will be discussed from a theoretical perspective, integrating research results that support clinical assessment approaches. Specific assessment tools will then be reviewed, highlighting the applicable age range, standard procedures and scope.

Feeding behavior

For oral feeding to result in adequate nutrition, the child must be an active participant. Behavior must support oral feeding, with the child awake, calm and cooperative for effective feeding. Children who are sleepy, agitated, or refusing to feed will generally not get adequate nutrition. While we know the importance of adequate nutrition, this may not be the motivating factor for the child. Typical motivators for feeding are pleasure from taste and sensation, social interaction, and the relief of hunger. Feeding refusal and other maladaptive behaviors may be observed if oral feeding is difficult for the child or if these underlying motivators are impaired.

While it is relatively easy to determine that a child's behavior is interfering with oral feeding, it may be more difficult to determine the root of this behavior. A variety of factors underlie behaviors which do not support feeding. These must be identified and resolved before programs to increase oral feeding will be successful. Such factors, and their associated behavioral and interactive patterns, are an important part of a feeding evaluation.

Factors contributing to abnormal feeding behavior
MEDICAL FACTORS
Feeding refusal in infants usually has an underlying physiological or medical cause. Primary medical factors to be considered include respiratory distress, swallowing dysfunction and pain from gastroesophageal reflux, with oral lesions and other sources of discomfort also potential contributors. Feeding refusal can result if the rate of fluid flow surpasses the infant's ability to coordinate sucking, swallowing and breathing, or if the infant loses motivation because sucking efforts have not been effective in alleviating hunger.

Feeding refusal in the older, neurologically disabled child can also be a consequence of underlying medical factors and not simply a manifestation of volitional behavior. For example, swallowing dysfunction leading to aspiration is a frequent problem in this population (Griggs et al. 1989, Morton et al. 1993, Rogers et al. 1994) and may lead to feeding refusal (Kenny et al. 1992). Long standing gastroesophageal reflux in the older child with cerebral palsy (Sondheimer and Morris 1979) and the resulting association between discomfort and eating can result in feeding refusal. Alternatively, previous medical problems that are now resolved, particularly pain from esophagitis, can lead to feeding refusal that is maintained on a behavioral basis alone.

Prior to implementing programs to increase oral feeding, therefore, it is crucial to ascertain that there are no current medical problems. Failure to do this can result in stronger patterns of feeding refusal, and can be potentially dangerous for the child who is aspirating.

AGITATION

Agitation during feeding may be part of the child's refusal behavior. Central nervous system abnormalities may result in an inability to filter sensory input and/or modulate responses to that input, so that reactions to feeding difficulties are magnified. Factors that produce stress or discomfort to the child can also lead to agitation. In young infants, for example, lack of adequate physical containment or support can produce stress and agitation (Als 1986). In tube-fed children agitation may be secondary to specific problems such as dumping syndrome or abdominal distention from gas bloat (Rossi 1993).

LETHARGY

Sleepiness and lethargy which interfere with feeding and intake often have a specific medical cause, *e.g.* hypoxia. Rogers *et al.* (1993*a*), for example, reported that lethargy improved when supplemental oxygen was provided during meal-times. In addition, the effect of medications should be considered when lethargy that interferes with feeding is observed (Rogers and Campbell 1993).

LEARNED AVERSION TO FEEDING

For a child who has always struggled with feeding, eating may not be a pleasurable experience. The sights, sounds, tastes and smells of feeding may become associated with the pain or discomfort of gastroesophageal reflux, inadequate ventilation, aspiration, or difficulty in satisfying hunger. In some cases, suppression of swallowing can occur (Walter 1994). The persistence of patterns of negative feeding behavior after removal of unpleasant stimuli is seen particularly in infants who have undergone long periods of unpleasant perioral stimulation from, for example, the use of endotracheal tubes, suctioning or nasogastric tubes.

COMMUNICATION PROBLEMS

In children with more severe disabilities, physical skills are typically limited and communication skills are often poor. Thus, such children may be given fewer choices regarding feeding than would be usual for their age. These factors, together with the high degree of dependency on caretakers, may lead to a significant degree of frustration in the disabled child. In consequence, children may develop a range of manipulative behaviors as a way of attempting to gain control during feeding.

FEEDING INTERACTIONS

Social interaction is an important component of the eating process, which should be enjoyable for both the child and the caregiver. Reilly and Skuse (1992) found that 75 per cent of mothers of children with cerebral palsy and oral-motor dysfunction did not enjoy mealtimes and revealed a lack of verbal interaction with the children during feeding, with resumption of verbal interaction after the meal. Decreased interaction may lead to dissatisfaction with eating on the child's part, or to the child's use of negative behaviors to elicit greater interaction with the feeder. Neither response is adaptive toward the goal of nutritional intake.

Motor behavior and physical functioning

Motor control of the head, trunk and extremities is crucial to oral feeding, and head and trunk control are prerequisites for attaining optimum oral-motor skill (Mueller 1972, Morris and Klein 1987). To achieve self-feeding, children need to develop coordinated use of the upper extremities for hand-to-mouth activity and skilled use of tools such as spoons, forks, knives and cups. Thus a comprehensive feeding assessment should address aspects of the child's general motor control.

The specific areas that require to be assessed include muscle tone, primitive reflex activity, postural control and symmetry, general movement and motor function during feeding, feeding position, and self-feeding skills.

Tone abnormalities, retained primitive reflexes and abnormal patterns of movement can have a direct effect on oral-motor function. Neck extension may impair tongue movements and make jaw closure difficult, affecting the ability to close the mouth and to chew (Morris and Klein 1987, Wolf and Glass 1992). Neck extension during feeding has also been linked to an increased risk of aspiration, due to both the difficulty of elevating the larynx for airway protection in this position and difficulty in pharyngeal clearance (Morton *et al.* 1993). In assessment, therefore, it is important to determine not only the presence of abnormal motor activity but also the degree to which this influences feeding skills.

Tactile responses

Feeding requires appropriate responses to oral tactile stimuli. Qualities of the bolus in terms of size, shape and consistency, and changes in these characteristics with oral manipulation, need to be appreciated by the child for efficient feeding. In the child with neurologic impairment, registration and perception of tactile stimuli are often faulty.

Behavioral responses to the sensory aspects of feeding
When the sensory system is functioning normally, feeding elicits the appropriate motor responses to handle food and saliva. Problems in perception of sensory inputs may lead to hyper- or hypoactive responses to the sensations of feeding, often mirroring the child's responses to sensory stimuli found throughout the rest of the body (Mueller 1972).

Thus a response may be of greater magnitude than expected for the type or amount of sensory stimulation. This could include turning away from food or struggling when feeding tools are brought to the mouth. The responses of the hypersensitive child may include total movement patterns or abnormal movement (Mueller 1972).

Similarly, a child may show less response to sensory stimuli than would be expected, *e.g.* a minimal response to placement of food in the mouth. Drooling may be an indication of poor tactile responsiveness, with the build-up of saliva in the mouth being an insufficient trigger for oral manipulation or swallowing. Weiss-Lambrou *et al.* (1989) demonstrated that children with cerebral palsy who drooled were more likely to have poor oral tactile skills than a group of children who did not drool. This suggests the need for careful evaluation of oral sensory perception in children who drool.

The effect of sensory input on oral-motor responses
The tactile and other sensory qualities of food play an important role in eliciting appropriate oral-motor sequences and swallowing. In normal children, Gisel (1991) found that food texture was related to the number of chewing cycles used and to the total length of time to eat. In the child with cerebral palsy, certain food textures can lead to an increase in abnormal oral patterns. In particular, as texture is increased, tongue and jaw thrust may become more predominant (Helfrich-Miller *et al.* 1986, Kramer and Eicher 1993, Morton *et al.* 1993, Rogers *et al.* 1994).

Oral-motor control
Abnormalities in oral-motor function and control are prevalent in children with neurologic impairment (Ottenbacher *et al.* 1983, Helfrich-Miller *et al.* 1986). In general, oral-motor skill is related to overall development, with those children who show the greatest neuromotor impairment also typically showing the greatest deficits in oral-motor skill. Severe oral dyspraxia, however, can occur in the absence of other significant motor impairment.

Children who have oral-motor dysfunction may take up to fifteen times longer to eat a given amount of food than a weight controlled peer (Gisel and Patrick 1988). Weight gain and growth are also poor (Krick and Van Duyn 1984). Since function in the oral phase sets the stage for an adequate pharyngeal swallow, oral-motor deficits can also lead to swallowing dysfunction and aspiration (Morton *et al.* 1993).

Specific oral-motor abnormalities
A number of common abnormal oral-motor patterns have been identified in children with neurologic impairment. These relate to function of the jaw, lips, and tongue.

JAW FUNCTION
Common problems seen in the child with neurologic impairment include: (1) lack of appropriate jaw closure, with the mouth open at rest and possibly during feeding; (2) tonic biting, or the tight closure of the jaw in response to a stimulus on or around the mouth; and (3) poor grading of movement, where mouth opening is often exaggerated during food presentation and oral manipulation. 16 of 20 children with cerebral palsy studied by Lespargot *et al.* (1993) generally had their mouths open in association with involuntary contraction of the submental musculature and difficulty relaxing the mouth-floor musculature.

LIP FUNCTION
Poor lip seal is the most prevalent observation of abnormal lip function. Griggs *et al.* (1989), studying severely disabled children, found that all had poor lip seal resulting in loss of food from the mouth. Lip seal is often related to jaw function, as wide jaw excursion and a mouth-open posture interfere with the ability to bring the lips together. Lespargot *et al.* (1993) also observed this relationship, noting both the open mouth posture and poor lip closure in

their sample of children with cerebral palsy, and observed that lip closure is important to the development of intraoral suction pressure used in swallowing.

The tongue is the primary structure involved in bolus control and manipulation, and its function is impaired in a large percentage of children with cerebral palsy (Helfrich-Miller 1986, Rogers *et al.* 1994). Tongue thrust, poor lateral movement, and lack of central grooving to channel a bolus are all features of the abnormal tongue control. Using ultrasound, Kenny *et al.* (1989*a*) found a lack of posterior tongue movement in children with cerebral palsy when compared to normal subjects. Abnormal tongue function may result in high oral transit times and piecemeal deglutition, such problems being reported in 70–90 per cent of children with severe cerebral palsy (Morton *et al.* 1993, Rogers *et al.* 1994).

The role of food texture
A variety of food textures need to be used in assessment of oral-motor function, recognizing that there is a developmental progression in acquiring strategies for coping with different textures (Gisel 1991). In general, liquids are the most difficult to handle, and this can lead to swallowing dysfunction and aspiration (Rogers *et al.* 1994). By contrast, solid textures can elicit chewing skills not seen with softer textures. However, in two studies (Helfrich-Miller *et al.* 1986, Griggs *et al.* 1989) aspiration was more prevalent in some children fed on thicker textured foods than on liquids. Feeding was felt to improve in these children when changed to a liquid diet. As there is no clear texture that is always associated with improved oral-motor and feeding function, each texture must be assessed for each individual patient.

Temporomandibular joint contracture
Recently the presence of contractures in the temporomandibular joint have been identified, and their role in feeding problems considered by Pelegano *et al.* (1994). They noted late onset feeding problems in a group of older children with spastic quadriplegic cerebral palsy, who had previously had adequate oral feeding skills. Studying these children they found the mandible to be retracted, posteriorly rotated, and with decreased range of motion when compared to normal controls. Hence, temporomandibular joint range of motion must also be included in a comprehensive feeding assessment in this population.

Swallowing
It is increasingly apparent that there is a high incidence of swallowing dysfunction in individuals with neurologic impairment. Multiple studies find some type of swallowing abnormality in almost all patients with severe neuromotor impairment (Helfrich-Miller *et al.* 1986, Griggs *et al.* 1989, Morton *et al.* 1993, Rogers *et al.* 1994). In these studies swallowing problems ranged from delayed initiation of the swallowing reflex to incomplete clearance of the bolus and frank aspiration. The incidence of swallowing dysfunction in children with less severe neurologic impairment is not as clear, but the potential complications of swallowing dysfunction are evident.

In studying a group of severely disabled children, Griggs *et al.* (1989) found that those who had the greatest swallowing impairment on video swallowing study were also the most poorly nourished, and this group also has an increased risk of respiratory complications (see Chapter 5). Thus, the evaluation of swallowing function is a crucial component of a feeding evaluation. A number of assessment techniques are available to the feeding specialist. These include clinical evaluation and cervical auscultation, described here, and imaging studies such as videofluoroscopic swallowing study (VFSS) and ultrasound, which are described in Chapter 8.

Clinical evaluation of swallowing
Clinical evaluation of swallowing can identify the functional components of the swallow and alert the feeding specialist to the need for a more detailed swallowing evaluation. Studies show that clinical evaluation is only 50–66 per cent accurate in determining the presence or absence of aspiration (Splaingard *et al.* 1988, Linden *et al.* 1993), so specific diagnosis of swallowing problems is typically not possible on clinical evaluation. The clinical evaluation, however, can provide information that maximizes the effectiveness of more sophisticated imaging studies such as VFSS (Wolf and Glass 1992, Linden *et al.* 1993, Palmer *et al.* 1993).

During the clinical evaluation of swallowing, the oral, pharyngeal and esophageal phases must be considered. The role of oral-motor control in setting up the timing and initiation of the pharyngeal swallow should be assessed. Observations that are indications for further evaluation of the pharyngeal phase of swallowing include the following.
• *Coughing and choking.* Coughing and choking during feeding are commonly associated with swallowing dysfunction (Tuchman 1989). In some cases, however, coughing may be elicited as foods or liquids enter the laryngeal vestibule but are not aspirated; rather, they may be effectively removed from the airway by a productive cough. In addition, coughing and choking may be due to an incoordination of swallowing and breathing, rather than frank swallowing dysfunction, particularly in the infant who is breast- or bottle-fed. On the other hand, silent aspiration with no cough or other external evidence is described (Linden *et al.* 1993), hence the absence of coughing during feeding does not ensure the presence of safe swallowing.
• *History of frequent respiratory infections.* When a child has a history of frequent unexplained upper respiratory infections, swallowing dysfunction should be considered, as detailed in Chapter 5.
• *Multiple swallows.* Frequently a child needs more than one swallow to process a bolus. Oral-motor dysfunction may lead to poor bolus control resulting in piecemeal release of the bolus into the pharynx and requiring multiple swallows to clear. Multiple swallows may also be an indication of poor pharyngeal clearance with residue remaining in the pharynx after the initial swallow.
• *Difficulty handling oral secretions and drooling.* Pharyngeal pooling of secretions and the need for suctioning of the airway may be indicative of significant swallowing dysfunction. Spontaneous drooling may also be an indication of impaired swallowing function. Children with cerebral palsy have less spontaneous swallowing than normal children,

and those who also drool, swallow spontaneously at a rate of only 45 per cent of normal (Sochaniwskyj *et al.* 1986).

• *Noisy breathing.* Wet, gurgly or congested sounding breathing that begins or exacerbates during feeding is strongly suggestive of swallowing dysfunction. Often these sounds result from poor pharyngeal clearance and residue, putting the child at risk for aspiration after the swallow (Logemann 1986). Nasal reflux during swallowing can also lead to wet or congested breath sounds, because the child is breathing through food residue in the nasopharynx.

Cervical auscultation
By using a microphone or stethoscope placed adjacent to the pharynx and larynx, the feeding specialist is able to listen to the sounds of swallowing and respiration (Vice *et al.* 1990, Takahashi *et al.* 1994). Acoustic changes in swallow sounds may be heard in association with difference in the physical character or size of bolus, abnormalities in pharyngeal transit of the bolus, or penetration of bolus into or through the larynx before, during or after the swallow. Excessive secretions in the pharynx, choking or stridor can also be heard. The acoustic sounds can be recorded simultaneously with tracings of heart rate, respiratory rate and oxygen saturation.

Reilly (1993) has used this model clinically to evaluate the feeding, swallowing and breathing coordination of normal children and children with cerebral palsy. This technique holds some promise for wider clinical application for the evaluation of swallowing. Although a stethoscope can provide some information regarding swallow sounds, more sophisticated equipment such as accelerometers or noise cancelling microphones should be used to hear properly the frequencies associated with swallow sounds (Vice *et al.* 1990).

Coordination of oral, respiratory and swallowing functions
Although feeding performance is typically associated with oral structure and function, the coordination of breathing with oral and swallowing functions can play a key role in feeding dysfunction. Oral function sets the stage for the timing and initiation of swallowing, while respiration ceases during each swallow. For safe and efficient feeding, oral, swallowing and respiratory functions must be coordinated, and assessment of this coordination must be included in the feeding evaluation. For infants, the traditional view has been that they could swallow and breathe simultaneously, thereby sparing themselves the task of coordinating the two actions. However, recent studies indicate that during feeding there is always a cessation of respiration during the infant's swallow (Wilson *et al.* 1981, Weber *et al.* 1986, Mathew and Bhatia 1989, Selley *et al.* 1990*a*, Bamford *et al.* 1992). This disruption of breathing lasts approximately 1 second (Wilson *et al.* 1981) and typically occurs after exhalation (Selley *et al.* 1990*a*). Due to the infant's rapid sucking rate, and thus the need for frequent swallowing, infants must have split-second timing between sucking, swallowing and breathing for efficient intake. In older children and adults, the need to suspend breathing during swallowing has long been appreciated, although it is only recently that the effect of impairment in this function in neurologically impaired children has been studied (Kenny *et al.* 1989*a*, McPherson *et al.* 1992, Casas *et al.* 1994).

Evaluation of coordination of sucking, swallowing and breathing in infancy

When evaluating these functions, the feeding specialist observes performance in each area individually, as well as their coordinated action. Evaluation of respiratory function includes the respiratory rate at rest and during feeding, and should include a subjective estimate of respiratory effort. The quality of respiratory sounds and rhythm should be noted. Physiologic changes such as oxygen desaturation, apnea, color change and/or bradycardia should also be noted as these may be an indication of incoordination.

A smooth and rhythmic pattern is the hallmark of well coordinated sucking, swallowing and breathing. By listening and watching for the placement of breaths during sucking, the length and frequency of sucking bursts and pauses, and the organization of sucking over the feeding period, the baby's sucking rhythm or pattern can be determined. Several abnormal sucking patterns have been described: short sucking bursts, disorganized sucking and feeding-induced apnea (Wolf and Glass 1992).

The short sucking burst pattern is characterized by sucking bursts of only two to four sucks followed by lengthy pauses to breathe. This type of pattern may be secondary to respiratory compromise, poor endurance or swallowing dysfunction. In the disorganized pattern there is an overall lack of rhythm and organization, with variability in the length of the bursts and pauses and an irregularity in the placement of the breaths within the sucking burst. This type of pattern may be secondary to neurobehavioral disorganization, sensory based feeding difficulties or central nervous system deficits that result in poor oral-motor control.

Feeding-induced apnea occurs when the baby takes five or more sucks without interspersing a breath. This can result in oxygen desaturation and possibly bradycardia (Mathew 1988). Often this pattern is maturational, since it is more typically observed in preterm infants (Shivpuri *et al.* 1983, Mathew *et al.* 1985, Mathew 1988). It may also be related to the rate of liquid flow. As the rate of liquid flow increases, the swallowing rate also increases. Since swallowing suppresses breathing, a high swallowing rate leaves little time available for breathing. The baby may respond by voluntarily suppressing respiration during sucking and swallowing to accommodate for this rapid flow.

Coordination of feeding, swallowing and breathing in childhood

In older children, the coordination of breathing with swallowing and feeding continues to play an important role in eating, and disruptions in this coordination are particularly noticeable in children with neurologic deficits. During tasks such as sipping or chewing, children with cerebral palsy show a variety of differences in coordinating respiratory, oral and swallowing function. Further details regarding these functions are outlined in Chapter 5.

McPherson *et al.* (1992) found that children with cerebral palsy had difficulty timing and sustaining respiration during feeding. In contrast with normal subjects, children with cerebral palsy tended to swallow at varying times within the respiratory cycle, including prior to inspiration. In addition, during continuous sip–swallows, children with cerebral palsy did not reach peak inspiration on the accompanying breaths. This could result in a gradual reduction in ventilation. These factors make it more likely that the child with cerebral palsy will need to inhale at a time when residue is present in the pharynx, thus increasing the risk of aspiration.

TABLE 6.1
Areas of feeding-related performance assessed by various feeding evaluations*

Evaluation instrument (reference)	Behavior	General motoric control	Tactile responses	Oral-motor skill and control	Swallowing	Respiratory function	Coordination of functions
Schedule for Oral Motor Assessment (SOMA) (Reilly et al. 1995)	+/–	+/–	+/–	+	+		
Clinical Feeding Evaluation of Infants (Wolf and Glass 1992)	+	+	+	+	+	+	+
Oral-Motor Feeding Rating Scale (Jelm 1990)		+/–	+/–	+	+/–	+/–	
Exeter Dysphagia Assessment Technique (EDAT) (Selley et al. 1990b)					+	+	+
Multidisciplinary Feeding Profile (Kenny et al. 1989b)		+	+	+	+	+	
Pre-feeding Skills (Morris and Klein 1987)	+	+	+	+	+	+	+
Neonatal Oral-motor Assessment Scale (NOMAS) (Braun and Palmer 1985)				+			+/–

*Key: + indicates this area is assessed by this evaluation; +/– indicates that this area receives slight emphasis in this evaluation.

In this group of children, ventilation may also be suppressed during oral preparation and manipulation of a food bolus, in addition to during swallowing (Kenny *et al.* 1989, McPherson *et al.* 1992, Reilly 1993, Casas *et al.* 1994). The alteration of breathing throughout all aspects of feeding can result in physiologic changes such as oxygen desaturation (Rogers *et al.* 1993*a*). Therefore, observations should be made regarding the regularity of breathing, prolonged respiratory pauses, gasping respirations and respiratory effort. If ventilation or the coordination of oral, swallowing and breathing functions is felt to be significantly impaired, assessment with oximetry should be used to assess the impact of these problems.

Overview of assessment tools

There are many assessment tools which have been specifically developed to provide a framework for the administration of a pediatric feeding assessment and the recording of observations. Seven of these published tools are briefly presented below and in Table 6.1, to allow comparison of their scope and procedures. This listing does not include informal checklists or protocols developed for use by individual centers.

• Schedule for Oral-Motor Assessment—SOMA (Reilly *et al.* 1995)

   Purpose: to rate objectively oral-motor skills and identify areas of dysfunction which could contribute to feeding difficulties.

   Age range: 8–24 months.

   Administration: utilizes standard equipment, food types and procedures during administration. 20 minutes to administer. Session is videotaped for later scoring.

   Scoring: 75–90 items are scored pass or fail for each of 6 food types administered. They fall into categories of jaw, lip and tongue movements, and reactivity, acceptance, initiation, food loss/drooling, sequencing and swallowing.

   Types of feeding assessed: liquid (by breast/bottle and/or spouted cup, regular cup and straw), spoon feeding of purée, semi-solid and solid, and finger feeding of biscuit and dried fruit.

   Comments: An abbreviated screening version is being developed with information on interpretation of scores. Reliability and validity studies have been done (Skuse *et al.* 1995).

• Clinical Feeding Evaluation of Infants (Wolf and Glass 1992)

   Purpose: to provide a structured method of data collection in 6 broad areas related to infant feeding, and to provide a format to utilize the information effectively in determining the need for further evaluation, or in management of feeding problems.

   Age range: infants feeding by bottle or breast, though some sections applicable to spoon feeding and cup drinking.

   Administration: observational during typical feeding by caretaker or therapist. Some modifications to normal feeding may be made during assessment.

   Scoring: performance is described or rated based on detailed descriptions of evaluation techniques and observations for each item. No summary scores are determined, but extensive information is provided on interpretation of observations.

   Types of feeding assessed: bottle, breast, or readiness for these skills.

- Oral-Motor Feeding Rating Scale (Jelm 1990)

  Purpose: to provide a concise format for obtaining and recording information during feeding assessment and to assist in decisions regarding feeding management.

  Age range: 1 year to adulthood.

  Administration: observations are made during a typical meal.

  Scoring: oral-motor movements are scored on a six point scale of normal to abnormal function. General information is given on features that would be considered normal or abnormal, but not on gradations within the rating system. Other areas are rated as 'problem' or 'no problem', or notes are taken on performance. There are no summary scores, or information on interpretation of findings.

  Types of feeding assessed: breast, bottle, spoon, cup, biting, chewing, straw drinking, as applicable.

- Exeter Dysphagia Assessment Technique—EDAT (Selley *et al.* 1990*b*)

  Purpose: a non-invasive method to quantify swallowing function to differentiate dysphagia due to sensory nerve, motor nerve or functional involvement.

  Age range: 2 years to adulthood (Parrot *et al.* 1992).

  Administration: specialized equipment used to document oral, respiratory and swallowing features during small sample of swallowing. Contact of the spoon to the lips is recorded from a specially adapted stainless steel spoon with contact sensor. The pattern of inspiration and expiration is measured via airflow through a nasal cannula. Swallow sounds are recorded by means of a self-supporting throat microphone.

  Scoring: visual inspection of the chart record, and computation of absolute values and percentages of specific swallowing and breathing components. Objective information can be obtained on the duration of oral and pharyngeal phases of swallow, and the pattern of respiration before and during swallowing.

  Types of feeding assessed: liquid from a spoon.

  Comments: Comparison data are provided from normal subjects and from subjects with a variety of motor and neuromuscular diagnoses.

- Multidisciplinary Feeding Profile (Kenny *et al.* 1989*b*)

  Purpose: to provide a statistically based protocol to quantitatively assess feeding skills in children who are severely motorically impaired and who are dependent feeders.

  Age range: subjects during test development were aged 6–18 years.

  Administration: done in a structured assessment which takes 30–45 minutes.

  Scoring: items are scored using various rating methods, which are described in a detailed test manual. A numeric value is assigned to most responses. Total scores and section scores can be obtained. No interpretation is given to various score values, though scores for a particular patient can be compared over time.

  Types of feeding assessed: spoon feeding, biting, chewing, cup drinking, straw drinking.

  Comments: Reliability studies have been done (Judd *et al.* 1989).

- Developmental Pre-feeding Checklist (Morris and Klein 1987)

  Purpose: to provide a structured method to qualitatively and quantitatively describe feeding performance, obtain historical information and identify abnormal oral patterns.

Age range: can be used with children of all ages, but the developmental skills assessed emerge between birth and 24 months.

Administration: observations are made of the child's most typical feeding performance. The assessment can occur over as many sessions as needed to insure that all aspects of feeding behavior have been observed.

Scoring: checklist and descriptive format. No summary score or developmental level is obtained.

Types of feeding assessed: bottle or breast, liquid by cup, semi-solids, solids.

Comments: Extremely detailed observation, with large number of skills observed. Feeding specialist has the option of observing feeding skills on a developmental continuum by age, or the developmental progression within specific skill areas.

- Neonatal Oral-Motor Assessment Scale (NOMAS) (Braun and Palmer 1985)

  Purpose: to determine the degree of feeding impairment present in infants with medical problems (including those associated with preterm birth), focusing on oral-motor function.

  Age range: infants who are bottle feeding.

  Administration: typical feeding given to infant by evaluator; focus is on tongue and jaw movements.

  Scoring: normal and abnormal characteristics of oral-motor function are rated on a point scale. Scores are summed, with total scores placing children in categories of normal, disorganized or dysfunctional feeders.

  Types of feeding assessed: bottle, along with non-nutritive sucking.

  Comments: Scoring has been revised and reliability and validity studies done by Case-Smith and colleagues (Case-Smith 1988, Case-Smith *et al.* 1989).

REFERENCES

Als, H. (1986) 'A synactive model of neonatal behavioral organization: framework for the assessment of neuro-behavioral development in the premature infant and for support of infants and parents in the neonatal intensive care environment.' *Physical and Occupational Therapy in Pediatrics*, **6**, 3–53.

Arvedson, J.C., Brodsky, L. (1993) *Pediatric Swallowing and Feeding: Assessment and Management.* San Diego, CA: Singular Publishing.

Bamford, O., Taciak V., Gewolb, I.H. (1992) 'The relationship between rhythmic swallowing and breathing during suckle feeding in term neonates.' *Pediatric Research*, **31**, 619–624.

Bax, M. (1989) 'Eating is important.' *Developmental Medicine and Child Neurology*, **31**, 285–286. *(Editorial.)*

Braun, M.A., Palmer, M.M. (1985) 'A pilot study of oral-motor dysfunction in "at-risk" infants.' *Physical and Occupational Therapy in Pediatrics*, **5**, 13–25.

Casas. M.T., Kenny, D.J., McPherson, K.A. (1994) 'Swallowing/ventilation interactions during oral swallow in normal children and children with cerebral palsy.' *Dysphagia*, **9**, 40–46.

Case-Smith, J.C. (1988) 'An efficacy study of occupational therapy with high-risk neonates,' *American Journal of Occupational Therapy*, **42**, 499–506.

—— Cooper, P., Scala, V. (1989) 'Feeding efficiency of premature neonates,' *American Journal of Occupational Therapy*, **43**, 245–250.

Gisel, E.G. (1991) 'Effect of food texture on the development of chewing of children between six months and two years of age.' *Developmental Medicine and Child Neurology*, **33**, 69–79.

—— Patrick, J. (1988) 'Identification of children with cerebral palsy unable to maintain a normal nutritional state.' *Lancet*, **1**, 283–286.

Glass, R.P., Wolf, L.S. (1993) 'Feeding and oral-motor skills.' *In:* Case-Smith, J. (Ed.) *Pediatric Occupational Therapy and Early Intervention.* Boston: Andover Medical, pp. 225–288.

Griggs, C.A., Jones, P.M., Lee, R.E. (1989) 'Videofluoroscopic investigation of feeding disorders of children with multiple handicap.' *Developmental Medicine and Child Neurology*, **31**, 303–308.

Helfrich-Miller, K.R., Rector, K.L., Straka, J.A. (1986) 'Dysphagia: its treatment in the profoundly retarded patient with cerebral palsy.' *Archives of Physical Medicine and Rehabilitation*, **67**, 520–525.

Jelm, J.M. (1990) *Oral-Motor/Feeding Rating Scale*. Tucson, AZ: Therapy Skill Builders.

Jones, P.M. (1989) 'Feeding disorders in children with multiple handicaps.' *Developmental Medicine and Child Neurology*, **31**, 404–406.

Judd, P.L., Kenny, D.J., Koheil, R., Milner, M., Moran, R. (1989) 'The multidisciplinary feeding profile: a statistically based protocol for assessment of dependent feeders.' *Dysphagia*, **4**, 29–34.

Kenny, D.J., Casas, M.J., McPherson, K.A. (1989a) 'Correlation of ultrasound imaging of oral swallow with ventilatory alterations in cerebral palsied and normal children: preliminary observations,' *Dysphagia*, **4**, 112–117.

—— Koheil, R.M., Greenberg, J., Reid, D., Milner, M., Moran, R., Judd, P.L. (1989b) ' Development of a multidisciplinary feeding profile for children who are dependent feeders,' *Dysphagia*, **4**, 16–28.

—— McPherson, K.A., Casas, M.J., Judd, P.L. (1992) 'Clinical Applications of Feeding Research.' *Paper presented at the Annual Meeting of the American Academy for Cerebral Palsy and Developmental Medicine, San Diego, CA.*

Kramer, S.S., Eicher, P.M. (1993) 'The evaluation of pediatric feeding abnormalities.' *Dysphagia*, **8**, 215–224.

Krick, J., Van Duyn, M.A.S. (1984) 'The relationship between oral-motor involvement and growth: a pilot study in a pediatric population with cerebral palsy.' *Journal of the American Dietetic Association*, **84**, 555–559.

Lefton-Greif, M.A. (1994) 'Diagnosis and management of pediatric feeding and swallowing disorders: role of the speech–language pathologist.' *In:* Tuchman, D.N., Walter, R.S. (Eds.) *Disorders of Feeding and Swallowing in Infants and Children: Pathophysiology, Diagnosis and Treatment.* San Diego, CA: Singular Publishing, pp. 97–114.

Lespargot, A., Langevein, M-F., Muller, S., Guillemont, S. (1993) 'Swallowing disturbances associated with drooling in cerebral-palsied children.' *Developmental Medicine and Child Neurology*, **35**, 298–304.

Linden, P., Kuhlemeier, K.V., Patterson, C. (1993) 'The probability of correctly predicting subglottic penetration from clinical observations.' *Dysphagia*, **8**, 170–179.

Logemann, J. (1986) 'Treatment for aspiration related to dysphagia: an overview.' *Dysphagia*, **1**, 43–48.

Mathew, O. P. (1988) 'Respiratory control during nipple feeding in preterm infants.' *Pediatric Pulmonology*, **5**, 220–224.

—— Bhatia, J. (1989) 'Sucking and breathing patterns during breast- and bottle-feeding in term neonates. Effects of nutrient delivery and composition.' *American Journal of Diseases of Children*, **143**, 588–592.

—— Clark, M.L., Pronske, M.L., Luna-Solarzano, H.G., Peterson, M.D. (1985) 'Breathing pattern and ventilation during oral feeding in term newborn infants.' *Journal of Pediatrics*, **106**, 810–813.

McPherson, K. A., Kenny, D.J., Koheil, R., Bablich, K., Sochaniwskyj, A., Milner, M. (1992) 'Ventilation and swallowing interactions of normal children and children with cerebral palsy.' *Developmental Medicine and Child Neurology*, **34**, 577–588.

Morris, S.E., Klein, M.D. (1987) *Pre-feeding Skills*. Tucson, AZ: Therapy Skill Builders.

Morton, R.E., Bonas, R., Fourie, B., Minford, J. (1993) 'Videofluoroscopy in the assessment of feeding disorders of chilren with neurological problems.' *Developmental Medicine and Child Neurology*, **35**, 388–395.

Mueller, H. (1972) 'Facilitating feeding and prespeech.' *In:* Pearson, P.H., Williams, C.E. (Eds.) *Physical Therapy Services in the Developmental Disabilities*. Springfield, IL: Charles C. Thomas, pp. 283–310.

Nwaobi, O.M., Smith, P.D. (1986) 'Effect of adaptive seating on pulmonary function of children with cerebral palsy,' *Developmental Medicine and Child Neurology*, **28**, 351–354.

Ottenbacher, K., Bundy, A., Short, M.A. (1983) 'The development and treatment of oral-motor dysfuction: a review of clinical research.' *Physical and Occupational Therapy in Pediatrics*, **3**, 1–13.

Palmer, J. B.,Kuhlemeier, K.V., Tippett, D.C., Lynch, C. (1993) 'A protocol for the videofluorographic swallowing study.' *Dysphagia*, **8**, 209–214.

Parrott, L.C., Selley, W.G., Brooks, W.A., Lethbridge, P.C., Cole, J.J., Flack, F.C., Ellis, R.E., Phil, M., Tripp, J.H. (1992) 'Dysphagia in cerebral palsy: a comparative study of the Exeter dysphagia assessment technique and a multidisciplinary assessment.' *Dysphagia*, **7**, 209–219.

Pelegano, J.P., Nowysz, S., Goepferd, S. (1994) 'Temporomandibular joint contracture in spastic quadriplegia: effect on oral-motor skills.' *Developmental Medicine and Child Neurology*, **36**, 487–494.

60

Reilly, S. (1993) 'The use of cervical auscultation in evaluation and therapy of oral and pharyngeal dysphagia.' *Paper presented at the Annual Meeting of the American Academy for Cerebral Palsy and Developmental Medicine, Nashville, TN.*

—— Skuse, D. (1992) 'Characteristics and management of feeding problems of young children with cerebral palsy.' *Developmental Medicine and Child Neurology*, **34**, 379–388.

—— Carroll, L., Barnett, S. (1993) Videofluroscopy in the assessment of feeding disorders.' *Developmental Medicine and Child Neurology*, **35**, 932–933. *(Letter.)*

—— Skuse, D., Mathisen, B., Wolke, D. (1995) 'The objective rating of oral-motor functions during feeding.' *Dysphagia*, **10**, 177–191.

Rogers, B., Campbell, J. (1993) 'Pediatric Neurodevelopmental Evaluation.' *In:* Arvedson, J.C., Brodsky, L. (Eds.) *Pediatric Swallowing and Feeding: Assessment and Management.* San Diego, CA: Singular Publishing, pp. 53–92.

—— Arvedson, J., Msall, M., Demerath, R.R. (1993a) 'Hypoxemia during oral feeding of children with severe cerebral palsy.' *Developmental Medicine and Child Neurology*, **35**, 3–10.

—— Msall, M., Shucard, D. (1993b) 'Hypoxemia during oral feedings in adults with dysphagia and severe neurological disabilities.' *Dysphagia*, **8**, 43–48.

—— Arvedson, J., Buck, G., Smart, P., Msall, M. (1994) 'Characteristics of dysphagia in children with cerebral palsy.' *Dysphagia*, **9**, 69–73.

Rossi, T. (1993) 'Pediatric gastroenterology,' *In:* Arvedson, J.C., Brodsky, L. (Eds.) *Pediatric Swallowing and Feeding: Assessment and Management.* San Diego, CA: Singular Publishing, pp. 123–156.

Selley, W. G., Ellis, R.E., Flack, F.C., Brooks, W.A. (1990a) 'Coordination of sucking, swallowing and breathing in the newborn: its relationship to infant feeding and normal development.' *British Journal of Disorders of Communication*, **25**, 311–327.

—— Flack, F.C., Ellis, R.E., Brooks, W.A. (1990b) 'The Exeter Dysphagia Assessment Technique.' *Dysphagia*, **4**, 227–235.

Shivpuri C. R., Martin, R.J., Carlo, W.A., Fanaroff, A.A. (1983) 'Decreased ventilation in preterm infants during oral feeding.' *Journal of Pediatrics*, **103**, 285–289.

Skuse, D., Stevenson, J., Reilly, S., Mathisen, B. (1995) 'Schedule for oral motor assessment (SOMA): methods of validation.' *Dysphagia*, **10**, 192–202.

Sochaniwskyj, A.E., Mother, R., Koheil, R., Bablich, K., Milner, M., Kenny, D.J. (1986) 'Oral motor functioning, frequency of swallowing and drooling in normal children and in children with cerebral palsy.' *Archives of Physical Medicine and Rehabilitation*, **67**, 866–874.

Sondheimer, J.M., Morris, B.A. (1979) 'Gastroesophageal reflux among severely retarded children,' *Journal of Pediatrics*, **94**, 710–714.

Splaingard, M.L., Hutchins, B., Sulton, L.D., Chaudhuri, G. (1988) ' Aspiration in rehabilitation patients: videofluoroscopy vs bedside clinical assessment,' *Archives of Physical Medicine and Rehabilitation*, **69**, 637–640.

Takahashi, K., Groher, M.E., Michi, K. (1994) 'Methodology for detecting swallowing sounds.' *Dysphagia*, **9**, 54–62.

Tuchman, D. N. (1989) 'Cough, choke, sputter: the evaluation of the child with dysfunctional swallowing.' *Dysphagia*, **3**, 111–116.

—— Walter, R.S. (1994) *Disorders of Feeding and Swallowing in Infants and Children: Pathophysiology, Diagnosis and Treatment.* San Diego, CA: Singular Publishing.

Vice, F.L., Heinz, J.M., Giuriati, G., Hood, M., Bosma, J.F. (1990) 'Cervical auscultation of suckle feeding in newborn infants.' *Developmental Medicine Child and Neurology*, **32**, 760–768.

Walter, R.S. (1994) 'Issues surrounding the development of feeding and swallowing.' *In:* Tuchman, D.N., Walter, R.S. (Eds.) *Disorders of Feeding and Swallowing in Infants and Children: Pathophysiology, Diagnosis and Treatment.* San Diego, CA: Singular Publishing, pp. 27–36.

Weber, F., Woolridge, M.W., Baum, J.D. (1986) 'An ultrasonographic study of the organisation of sucking and swallowing by newborn infants.' *Developmental Medicine and Child Neurology*, **28**, 19–24.

Weiss-Lambrou, R., Tétreault, S., Dudley, J. (1989) 'The relationship between oral sensation and drooling in persons with cerebral palsy.' *American Journal of Occupational Therapy*, **43**, 155–161.

Wilson, S. L., Thack, B.T., Brouillette, R.T., Abu-Osba Y.K. (1981) 'Coordination of breathing and swallowing in human infants.' *Journal of Applied Physiology*, **50**, 851–858.

Wolf, L.S., Glass, R.G. (1992) *Feeding and Swallowing Disorders in Infancy: Assessment and Management.* Tucson, AZ: Therapy Skill Builders.

7
NUTRITIONAL ASSESSMENT OF THE DISABLED CHILD

Virginia A. Stallings and Babette S. Zemel

Importance of nutritional assessment

There is insufficient information on nutritional needs or nutritional status of children with severe disabilities to make clear recommendations for nutrient intake and growth pattern expectations. Neurologic abnormalities result in altered physical activity (voluntary and involuntary), fine motor and oral-motor patterns. These alterations create a high level of risk for malnutrition by affecting food intake and nutrient requirements. Nutritional status assessment is the process by which the medical care team identifies which individual patient is under- or overnourished. Nutritional assessment of children with moderate to severe disabilities is complicated by the interactions of the primary disease process (*e.g.* muscle atrophy, contractures, spasticity, central nervous system pathology) and both chronic and acute malnutrition. Cerebral palsy (CP), a common disability with significant risk for malnutrition, will be the clinical example for this discussion of nutritional assessment of children with disabilities.

Nutritional assessment in children with CP requires evaluation of dietary intake, growth, body composition and laboratory data in the context of the nutritional risk factors related to the medical history, diagnosis and current therapy. Investigators have provided some information on these topics over the past 40 years. Many of the findings are limited by small sample sizes and changes in therapeutic approaches when compared to contemporary standards of care. Yet, a pattern of inadequate food intake, growth failure and disease-specific nutritional concerns is apparent.

Early studies of food intake, nutritional status, growth, body composition and nutritional biochemical measurements of children with CP were conducted and reported by several investigators (Peeks and Lamb 1951, Phelps 1951, Leamy 1953, Sterling 1960, Karle *et al.* 1961, Tobis *et al.* 1961, Ruby and Matheny 1962, Culley *et al.* 1963, Hammond *et al.* 1966, Pryor and Thelander 1967, Berg and Isaksson 1970). As was common until the early 1970s, most of these children were in large residential institutions. This body of work was the basis of recognition of several important nutritional themes for children with CP, including: food intake low in calories and occasionally low in selected nutrients, including vitamins C, A, D and iron and calcium; marked linear growth failure and poor weight gain; abnormal body composition with changes in the muscle and fat stores; and significant occurrence of undernutrition (failure to thrive, marasmus) and less frequently overnutrition (overweight, obesity).

In the 1970s, research interest turned to recognizing the drug–nutrient interaction of anticonvulsant medications and vitamin D metabolism. Anticonvulsants, through action of the hepatic microsomal enzymes, cause increased vitamin D catabolism. This, combined with low dietary intake of vitamin D and calcium, and low sunlight exposure for vitamin D, resulted in rickets, osteopenia and pathological fractures in some children with CP (Lifshitz and Maclaren 1973, Crosley et al. 1975, Tolman et al. 1975, Mimaki et al. 1980).

Over the last decade many nutrition and developmental disabilities issues have been investigated. The relationship of oral-motor dysfunction, food intake and growth has been explored by several investigators (Krick and Van Duyn 1984; Gisel and Patrick 1988; Thommessen et al. 1991a,b,c; Croft 1992; Reilly and Skuse 1992; Dahl and Gebre-Medhin 1993), and is discussed in several chapters of this volume. The need for interdisciplinary evaluation and treatment of nutrition and feeding abnormalities for children and adults with CP has been addressed by investigators and position papers (Johnson and Maeda 1989, Wodarski 1990, Boyle 1991, Blyler and Lucas 1992, Ferrang et al. 1992). In addition, several nutrition intervention trials with caloric supplementation by gastrostomy or naso-gastric feeding tube have shown improvements of various components of nutritional status in children with CP (Patrick et al. 1986, Shapiro et al. 1986, Rempel et al. 1988, Sanders et al. 1990, Fried and Pencharz 1991).

In an effort to identify the nutritional component of growth failure in spastic quadri-plegic CP, Stallings et al. (1993a) assessed 142 children aged 2–18 years. Mean upper-arm and lower-leg lengths were found to be significantly reduced (z scores −1.57 to −2.38) relative to age- and sex-specific reference norms for healthy children (Spender et al. 1989). Mean body weight and triceps skinfold thickness were reduced to about 65 per cent of the median and subscapular skinfold fat stores to 81 per cent of the median for US children. Examination of the sample showed reduction in growth and nutritional status indicators even in children as young as 2–4 years. To determine more clearly the degree to which nutri-tional status affected linear growth, a set of two-step regression analyses was conducted. The linear growth measures were significantly correlated with measures of nutritional status (arm muscle area, percentage of body fat), after controlling for disease severity (diagnosis, cognitive ability, oral-motor function, ambulatory status, gastrostomy feeding and dyskinetic component) and non-disease variables (age, gender, race, pubertal status, parental height). In other words, poor nutritional status had an effect on linear growth that was independent of and additional to the effects of disease severity and non-disease factors.

A similar study of 154 children with diplegic or hemiplegic CP showed reduced linear growth compared to the norms for healthy children (Stallings et al. 1993b). About 30 per cent of the sample was undernourished, indicated by low body weight for age or depleted fat stores at the triceps skinfold site. 8–14 per cent were overweight, depending on the cri-teria used. Children in the youngest age group were the most at-risk for poor nutritional status and delayed growth.

Nutritional status assessment
Inadequate caloric intake appears to be a major cause of nutrition-related growth failure in children with CP. Thus, two clinical management needs arise: (1) methods to assess nutri-tional and growth status to identify patients who are undernourished (too few calories) or

TABLE 7.1
Clinical signs of nutritional deficiency

Sign	Nutrient
General	
Weight	Acute protein–calorie malnutrition (PCM)
Height	Chronic PCM, zinc, protein
Head circumference	Chronic PCM
Skin	
Pallor	Iron, folate, copper, vitamins B_6, B_{12}
Petechiae, purpura	Vitamins C, K
Seborrheic dermatitis	Vitamin B_6, riboflavin, zinc
Dryness, xerosis	Zinc, vitamin A, biotin, essential fatty acid (linoleic acid)
Follicular keratosis	Vitamin A
Pellagrous dermatosis	Niacin, tryptophan
Hair	
Alopecia	Protein, zinc
Hypopigmentation, brittle	Protein, biotin
Eyebrow loss	Biotin
Glands	
Goiter	Iodine
Parotid enlargement	Acute or chronic PCM
Nails	
Koilonychia	Iron
Chest	
Pigeon breast, rachitic rosary	Vitamin D
Cardiac	
Tachycardia	Iron, thiamin
Congestive heart failure, cardiomegaly	Thiamin, selenium
Arrhythmia	Magnesium, potassium, calcium
Abdomen	
Hepatomegaly	Protein, chronic PCM
Ascites, protuberant	Protein
Extremities	
Muscle wasting	Acute or chronic PCM
Peripheral oedema	Protein, thiamin
Malleolar splaying, bowed-leg	Vitamin D
Neurological	
Mental confusion, irritability	Niacin, thiamin, vitamin B_{12}
Decreased position or vibration sense	Vitamin B_{12}, riboflavin
Ataxia, loss of ankle and knee reflexes	Vitamins B_1, B_{12}, E, thiamin, calcium, magnesium
Peripheral neuropathy	Vitamin B_6, thiamin

overnourished (too many calories); and (2) methods to determine the caloric requirement of the individual patient.

The elements of complete nutritional assessment are based on the standard pediatric medical evaluation, as follows.

The *medical history* includes assessment of the acute and chronic medical problems and medications. In addition, a nutritional history including review of a 'typical' day's

TABLE 7.2
Drug–nutrient interactions

Drug	Nutrient affected
Anticonvulsants	
Phenytoin	Folate, vitamins B_{12}, B_6, D, C, calcium
Phenobarbitone	Folate, vitamins B_{12}, B_6, K, C, calcium
Anti-inflammatory agents	
Aspirin	Vitamin C, iron
Corticosteroids	Protein, fat, zinc, sodium, potassium, calcium, glucose
Antimicrobials	
Isoniazid	Vitamin B_6, niacin
Trimethoprim	Folate
Penicillin	Potassium
Cathartics	
Mineral oil	Vitamins A, D, E, K, carotene, calcium
Others	
Digitalis	Potassium, magnesium, calcium
Frusemide	Zinc, calcium, sodium, potassium
Antacids	Phosphate, calcium, vitamin A, iron
Cholestyramine	Vitamins A, D, E, K, calcium, fat

food intake, past nutritional history, use of caloric, vitamin or mineral supplements, and unusual food practices by the child or family should be obtained. The past growth patterns, including pubertal onset and growth charts, are reviewed. The history would include a review of systems with emphasis on the dental and oral-motor function, and the gastrointestinal tract (emesis, gastroesophageal reflux, diarrhea, constipation).

The *physical examination* includes current weight, height or length or alternative linear growth measures, head circumference, mid-arm circumference, and skinfold measurements. Details of the recommended methods, equipment and reference standards for the anthropometric measurements are given in the following section. Table 7.1 provides an overview of the physical examination findings of nutritional deficiencies.

The *laboratory evaluation* is focused by recognizing the risk factors identified from the history and physical examination for each individual patient. The primary nutritional problem is usually inadequate caloric intake, and laboratory assessment of this pattern of malnutrition is limited. Both serum albumin and pre-albumin are indicators of the adequacy of calorie and protein intake, with albumin (half-life ~14–20 days) reflecting the last month's and pre-albumin (half-life ~2–3 days) reflecting the last week's nutrient intake. Iron deficiency anaemia is seen in groups of patients who have limited caloric intake or who have monotonous food intake with little meat or iron-rich vegetables. Iron status evaluation includes a complete blood count (hemoglobin, hematocrit, red cell indices) as a screen, followed by other iron studies (serum iron, total iron-binding capacity, transferrin, ferritin) as indicated. Response to iron therapy is monitored by changes in the components of the complete blood count and a reticulocyte count.

Laboratory tests depend upon the patient's history and may include serum values for vitamin D, calcium, phosphorous and alkaline phosphatase, and radiologic examination of long bones to diagnose rickets. Osteopenia can occur without rachitic changes and would be diagnosed by determining bone mineral content or bone density (single or dual photon absorptiometry, dual energy X-ray absorptiometry). Blood values for selected vitamins and minerals are available when indicated for selected patients. Table 7.2 summarizes common drug–nutrient interactions.

Anthropometry

Anthropometric assessment is a rapid and inexpensive means of determining short and long term nutritional status. Although these measures are non-invasive and can be accomplished with simple tools, they require a trained anthropometrist in order to ensure accurate, reproducible measurements. Numerous anthropometric measures are used in the assessment of nutritional status, since no single measure is sufficient for full characterization. Proper equipment should be used, and it should be checked regularly for accuracy. When anthropometric measurements are obtained under these conditions and compared to appropriate reference standards, the clinician is able to determine the current classification of nutritional status and perform periodic checks for changes in status. Guidelines for anthropometric measurement techniques are given by Cameron (1986) and Lohman *et al.* (1988).

Growth

Height or length and head circumference should be measured at routine visits. Measurement of growth by well-trained personnel using accurate equipment makes these measurements very informative, especially for tracking progress in individual patients.

WEIGHT

Because growth retardation is common, weight must be measured in conjunction with linear growth measures in order to distinguish between underweight and wasting. In addition, since excess weight can be caused by excess fat, excess lean or excess water (edema), it is essential to measure arm circumference and skinfold thicknesses in order to interpret a weight measurement. Weight increments are important for assessing changes in nutritional status.

Weight should be measured on a beam balance scale or a digital electronic scale. The scale should be checked weekly with known calibration weights. Weight of older children should be measured to the nearest 0.1 kg, and that of infants to the nearest 0.01 kg.

The scale should be set to zero before the child is placed on the scale. Weight measures should be taken with the child wearing little or no outer clothing and no shoes. Infants should be measured without diapers (nappies).

Reference standards have been published by Hamill *et al.* (1979), Roche and Himes (1980) and Guo *et al.* (1991).

LENGTH OR HEIGHT

Linear growth reflects the nutritional history of the patient and helps to distinguish between short and long term nutritional problems. When appropriate, a length or height measurement should be taken. Supine length measures are taken for children under the age of 2–3 years, and height is measured at age 2 or above. For children over 3 years of age who are not able to stand erect unsupported, a length measurement can be taken. However, when comparing this measurement to a growth chart for height, the length should be decreased by approximately 2 cm (see Roche and Davila 1974) to adjust for the known difference between length and height values due to gravity.

For length measurements, children should be measured on an infantometer or an inflexible length board with a fixed head board and a movable foot board.

Height should be measured by a stadiometer with a head paddle that glides smoothly but is firmly perpendicular to the back of the stadiometer. Alternatively, a tape measure permanently fixed to a wall or door frame can be used provided a head paddle is available that will fit at a 90° angle to the wall.

Length measurements require two people to position and hold the child. The head should be held firmly at the top of the board by an assistant, with the Frankfurt plane perpendicular to the floor. The Frankfurt plane extends from the lower margin of the orbit to the upper margin of the auditory meatus. The knees should be flattened firmly by the anthropometrist to fully extend the legs. The feet should be together and flexed to a 90° angle with the infant fully stretched. For height, the child should stand erect with the heels, buttocks and back of the head against the stadiometer. The heels should be placed together and the arms should be down and relaxed.

Both length and height measurements should be taken to the nearest 0.1 cm. Measurements should be taken in triplicate, with agreement within 0.5 cm, and the mean recorded.

Length and height measures are inappropriate for children with spinal curvature, contractures or any other condition that prevents proper positioning for the measurement. Upper arm length and lower leg length are alternatives under these conditions (see below). Proper positioning is the only way to ensure accurate, reproducible length measures so that linear growth increments can be incorporated into the nutritional component of clinical care.

Whenever possible, the heights of both biological parents should be obtained to compute mid-parental height (the average height of the mother and father). Adjustment of height or length measurements using mid-parental height charts (Himes *et al.* 1985) is a technique that recognizes and corrects for differences in the genetic potential for growth in height.

Reference standards have been published by Hamill *et al.* (1979), Roche and Himes (1980), Himes *et al.* (1985), Tanner and Davis (1985), Guo *et al.* (1991) and Berkey *et al.* (1993).

HEAD CIRCUMFERENCE

Because brain growth is most rapid in the first three years of life, head circumference should be included in the assessment of growth and nutritional status. Children with developmental disabilities often exhibit delayed or inadequate growth, so it is important to measure head circumference until age 3 (or longer in some children) to determine whether growth of the brain and head is also compromised.

A flexible metal or non-stretchable plastic-coated tape is used. Measuring tapes should be scaled to 0.1 cm. The tape should be placed superior to the supraorbital ridge and

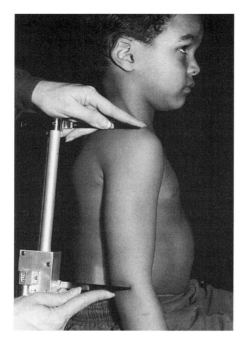
Fig. 7.1. Upper arm length measurement.

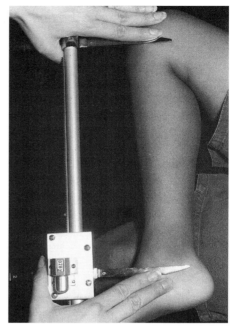
Fig. 7.2. Lower leg length measurement.

adjusted around the occiput until maximum circumference is obtained. The plane of the tape should be the same on both sides of the head, and care should be taken that the tape is evenly placed flat against the skull. The tape should be loosened and the head circumference re-measured so that three measurements are obtained, and the mean recorded. Hair pins and braids should be removed before measuring.

Reference standards have been published by Hamill *et al.* (1979), Roche and Himes (1980) and Roche *et al.* (1987).

UPPER ARM LENGTH AND LOWER LEG LENGTH

Length and height measurements frequently are not possible in children with developmental disabilities due to body shape abnormalities. Alternative measures are upper arm length and lower leg length which provide upper and lower body measures of long bone growth.

For young infants, sliding calipers (0–200 mm) can be used. For older infants and children, an anthropometer is used. All measurements should be taken in triplicate to the nearest 0.1 cm and repeated every 3 months.

For young children (0–24 months) upper arm length is measured as shoulder–elbow length, from the superior lateral surface of the acromion to the inferior surface of the elbow with the arm flexed at 90°. In children of 2–18 years, upper arm length is measured from

68

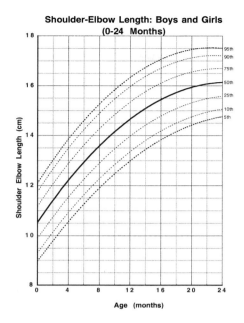

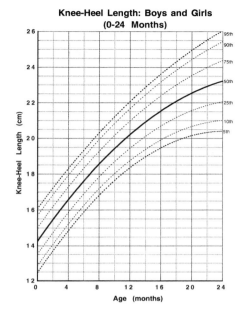

Fig. 7.3. Upper arm lengths for boys and girls aged 0–24 months.

Fig. 7.4. Lower leg lengths for boys and girls aged 0–24 months.

the superior lateral surface of the acromion to the head of the radius with the arm relaxed, as shown in Figure 7.1. In children below the age of 24 months, lower leg length is measured as knee–heel length from the heel to the superior surface of the knee. The infant should be lying on her back with the leg flexed to 90° at the hip, the knee and the ankle. For children aged 2–18 years, the lower leg length measure is taken from the lower border of the medial malleolus to the medial tip of the tibia, while the patient is sitting in a relaxed position as shown in Figure 7.2. Reference centiles for upper arm length and lower leg length for children aged 0–24 months are given in Figures 7.3–7.4; those for older children are shown in Figures 7.5–7.8*. For children with normal limb function bilaterally, or with dysfunction affecting both sides equally, the right side should be measured; otherwise, the least affected side should be measured and the side that is measured should be noted.

Reference standards have been published by Snyder *et al.* (1977) and Spender *et al.* (1989).

Nutritional status
Anthropometric indicators of nutritional status consist of circumferences and skinfold thicknesses at sites known to be sensitive to changes in nutrient intake and health. Upper arm

---

*Children aged 2–3 years should be plotted at the 3-year point for evaluation.

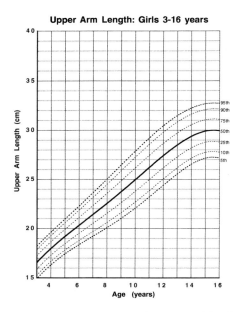

Fig. 7.5. Upper arm lengths for girls aged 3–16 years.

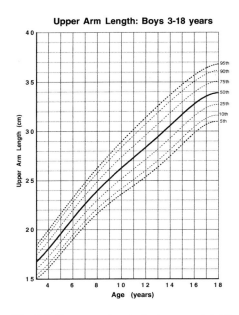

Fig. 7.6. Upper arm lengths for boys aged 3–18 years.

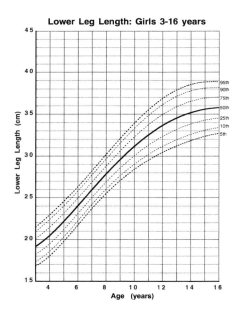

Fig. 7.7. Lower leg lengths for girls aged 3–16 years.

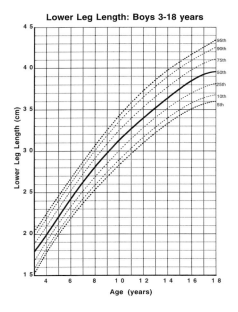

Fig. 7.8. Lower leg lengths for boys aged 3–18 years.

anthropometry is particularly useful because excellent reference data are available for interpretation of the measurements.

Upper arm circumference is a composite measure of muscle and fat stores at a site that is sensitive to current nutritional status.

Upper arm circumference is taken at the mid-point of the upper arm. The mid-point is located and marked by measuring the length of the upper arm (from the acromion to the olecranon with the arm flexed at 90°). The circumference is measured with the arm down in a fully relaxed position, with the tape measure perpendicular to the long axis of the arm. Measurements should be taken in triplicate to the nearest 0.1 cm, using a non-stretchable flexible tape. Care should be taken to ensure that the tape is neither too tight nor too loose. This guarantees that an accurate and reproducible measure is obtained.

Reference standards have been published by Frisancho (1981).

SKINFOLD THICKNESS

Skinfold thickness measures at the triceps and subscapular sites are indicators of whole body fat stores and are sensitive to changes in nutritional status. Depletion of fat stores at the triceps site is common in children with CP and other chronically undernourished groups (Spender *et al.* 1988), so measurement of two skinfolds is important for adequate characterization of body fat.

The triceps skinfold thickness is measured along the back of the arm, over the triceps muscle, at the same level where the mid-arm circumference is measured. The arm is down and fully relaxed for this measurement. The fold of fat and skin is lifted away from the underlying muscle at that site. The fold is held in position while the thickness is measured with calipers. Holtain skinfold calipers are preferred because they are scaled to 0.2 mm; Lange calipers can also be used, but with some loss of accuracy since they measure to the nearest 0.5 mm. The calipers are placed on the skin just below the fingers lifting up the fatfold, and the reading should be taken 4 seconds after releasing the caliper's handles.

An additional skinfold measurement should be taken at the subscapular site. The subscapular skinfold is an indicator of truncal fat stores. It is less sensitive to changes in short term nutritional status and a better reflection of long term status. The measurement is taken with the arm and shoulder down and fully relaxed. The fat fold is lifted 1 cm below the tip of the scapula at a downward angle following the natural contour of the body. As before, the calipers are placed next to the fingers holding the fold and the reading is taken 4 seconds after releasing the caliper handles.

Reference standards have been published by Frisancho (1981, 1990), Johnson *et al.* (1981) and Cronk and Roche (1982).

Body composition

Body composition is an essential component of nutritional assessment of the disabled child. Since linear growth is often affected, measurement of whole body fat stores and fat-free mass are important indicators of short term nutritional adequacy. For 8- to 18-year-olds,

TABLE 7.3

Anthropometric equations* for prediction of proportion of fat as percentage of body mass (ages 8–18 years)

White males
Prepubescent: 1.21 (triceps + subscapular) – 0.008 (triceps + subscapular)^2 – 1.7
Pubescent: 1.21 (triceps + subscapular) – 0.008 (triceps + subscapular)^2 – 3.4
Postpubescent: 1.21 (triceps + subscapular) – 0.008 (triceps + subscapular)^2 – 5.5

Black males
Prepubescent: 1.21 (triceps + subscapular) – 0.008 (triceps + subscapular)^2 – 3.2
Pubescent: 1.21 (triceps + subscapular) – 0.008 (triceps + subscapular)^2 – 5.2
Postpubescent: 1.21 (triceps + subscapular) – 0.008 (triceps + subscapular)^2 – 6.8

All females   1.33 (triceps + subscapular) – 0.013 (triceps + subscapular)^2 – 2.5

If (triceps + subscapular) >35 mm
Males: 0.783 (triceps + subscapular) + 1.6
Females: 0.546 (triceps + subscapular) + 9.7

*Triceps and subscapular skinfold thicknesses measured in millimetres. (Reproduced by permission from Slaughter *et al.* 1988.)

body composition can be determined using the anthropometric prediction equations of Slaughter *et al.* (1988). These equations use the triceps and subscapular skinfold measures and are specific to puberty status, gender and race, as shown in Table 7.3.

In children with spastic quadriplegic CP, the Slaughter prediction equations for fat mass have been found to be significantly correlated ($r=0.69$) with measures of fat mass determined from stable isotopes (Stallings, unpublished). Bioelectrical methods such as total body electrical conductivity (TOBEC) and bioelectrical impedance analysis (BIA) are feasible but may be subject to increased measurement error due to motion artifact in children with spasticity. In addition, both TOBEC and BIA methodologies require a height measurement, rendering them less effective in children whose actual height can only be estimated from long bone measures.

Reference standards have been published by Fomon *et al.* (1982), Slaughter *et al.* (1988) and Frisancho (1990).

Energy recommendations

Assessment of energy intake compared to requirement is an essential component of the nutritional care of children with significant disabilities. Undernutrition and overnutrition are the common nutritional pathologies and are the result of energy imbalance. True energy intake is often difficult to determine accurately in children with poor oral-motor function and other gastrointestinal problems. Daily energy expenditure and its components can be measured in individuals in a research setting (doubly labelled water, 24-hour indirect room calorimetry, resting energy expenditure, thermic effect of food, physical activity). Only resting energy expenditure, a measurement of basal metabolic needs, can be evaluated clinically, and can be used with estimates of physical activity to predict total caloric needs.

The use of population standards for energy recommendation, such as the Recommended Dietary Allowance from the USA, are not helpful for individual patients with atypical body

TABLE 7.4
**Equations for predicting resting energy expenditure
from body weight (in kg) (W)***

Age (y)	Male	Female
0–3	60.9 W − 54	61.0 W − 51
3–10	22.7 W + 495	22.5 W + 499
10–18	17.5 W + 651	12.2 W + 746
18–30	15.3 W + 679	14.7 W + 496
30–60	11.6 W + 879	8.7 W + 829
>60	13.5 W + 487	10.5 W + 596

*Adapted from data published by WHO (1985).

size, body composition and physical activity. The formulas for energy requirement from the World Health Organization (WHO 1985) are more useful and allow for more individualized prediction of resting energy expenditure based on gender, age and body weight (Table 7.4). The value for resting energy expenditure is adjusted by an activity factor to determine total energy expenditure. In normally active, healthy children and adults with light or moderate activity, the activity factors range from 1.50 to 1.89 times the resting energy expenditure. Recent work by the present authors (unpublished) suggests that the physical activity factor for well-nourished children with spastic quadriplegia is much lower, about 1.3 times the resting energy expenditure, and for those who are malnourished, about 1.5 times.

Two other methods for estimating caloric requirements have been published. Culley and Middleton (1969) developed a method for mentally retarded children which takes level of motor function into account. Daily caloric consumption by this method was: 14.7 kcal/cm of height and 77 kcal/kg for children without motor dysfunction; 13.9 kcal/cm and 75 kcal/kg for ambulatory children with motor dysfunction; and 11.1 kcal/cm and 64 kcal/kg for non-ambulatory children with motor dysfunction. Krick *et al.* (1992) reported a factorial approach to determining caloric needs in children with CP. This method accounts for caloric intake based on: estimated resting energy expenditure needs; muscle-tone alterations; normal growth needs; and catch-up growth or nutritional repletion in malnourished children. The formula is summarized as: calories/day = (resting energy needs × tone factor × activity factor) + growth factor(s).

Summary
Nutrition and growth status in children and adults with CP and other severe types of developmental disabilities is an essential component of care. While data are not available to provide precise definitions of the levels of severity of malnutrition and growth failure and their effect on long-term outcome, it is clear that many patients with moderate and severe CP and other disabilities have malnutrition and growth failure as the result of inadequate caloric intake. Nutritional status assessment every 3–6 months will enable the clinical care team to identify malnutrition and growth failure, and provide an objective means of following the response to nutritional intervention.

ACKNOWLEDGEMENTS

Supported in part by the United Cerebral Palsy Foundation, the Cystic Fibrosis Foundation, the General Clinical Research Center (NIH-RR-00240), and the Nutrition Center of The Children's Hospital of Philadelphia.

REFERENCES

Berg, K., Isaksson, B. (1970) 'Body composition and nutrition of school children with cerebral palsy.' *Acta Paediatrica Scandanavica*, Suppl. 204, 41–52.

—— Olsson, T. (1970) 'Energy requirements of school children with cerebral palsy as determined from indirect calorimetry.' *Acta Paediatrica Scandanavica*, Suppl. 24, 71–80.

Berkey, C.S., Dockery, D.W., Wang, X., Wypij, D., Ferris, B. (1993) 'Longitudinal height velocity standards for U.S. adolescents.' *Statistics in Medicine*, **12**, 403–414.

Blyler, E.M., Lucas, B.L. (1992) 'Position of the American Dietetic Association: nutrition in comprehensive program planning for persons with developmental disabilities.' *Journal of the American Dietetic Association*, **92**, 613–615.

Boyle, J.T. (1991) 'Nutritional management of the developmentally disabled child.' *Pediatric Surgery International*, **6**, 76–81.

Cameron, N. (1986) 'The methods of auxological anthropology.' *In:* Falkner, F., Tanner, J.M. (Eds.) *Human Growth: a Comprehensive Treatise, 2nd Edn, Vol. 3*. New York, Plenum Press, pp. 3–46.

Croft, R.D. (1992) 'What consistency of food is best for children with cerebral palsy who cannot chew?' *Archives of Disease in Childhood*, **67**, 269–271.

Cronk, C.E., Roche, A.F. (1982) 'Race- and sex-specific reference data for triceps and subscapular skinfolds and weight/stature^2.' *American Journal of Clinical Nutrition*, **35**, 347–354.

Crosley, C.J., Chee, C., Berman, P.H. (1975) 'Rickets associated with long-term anticonvulsant therapy in a pediatric outpatient population.' *Pediatrics*, **56**, 52–57.

Culley, W.J., Middleton, T.O. (1969) 'Caloric requirements of mentally retarded children with and without motor dysfunction.' *Journal of Pediatrics*, **75**, 380–384.

—— Jolly, D.H., Mertz, E.T. (1963) 'Heights and weights of mentally retarded children.' *American Journal of Mental Deficiency*, **68**, 203–210.

Dahl, M., Gebre-Medhin, M. (1993) 'Feeding and nutritional problems in children with cerebral palsy and myelomeningocoele.' *Acta Paediatrica Scandinavica*, **82**, 816–820.

Eddy, T.P., Nicholson, A.L., Wheeler, E.F. (1965) 'Energy expenditures and dietary intakes in cerebral palsy.' *Developmental Medicine and Child Neurology*, **7**, 377–386.

Ferrang, T.M., Johnson, R.K., Ferrara, M.S. (1992) 'Dietary and anthropometric assessment of adults with cerebral palsy.' *Journal of the American Dietetic Association*, **92**, 1083–1086.

Fomon, S.J., Haschke, F., Ziegler, E.E., Nelson, S.E. (1982) 'Body composition of reference children from birth to age 10 years.' *American Journal of Clinical Nutrition*, **35**, 1169–1175.

Fried, M.D., Pencharz, P.B. (1991) 'Energy and nutrient intakes of children with spastic quadriplegia.' *Journal of Pediatrics*, **119**, 947–949.

Frisancho, A.R. (1981) 'New norms of upper limb fat and muscle areas for assessment of nutritional status.' *American Journal of Clinical Nutrition*, **34**, 2540–2545.

—— (1990) *Anthropometric Standards for the Assessment of Growth and Nutritional Status.* Ann Arbor, MI: University of Michigan Press.

Gisel, E.G., Patrick, J. (1988) 'Identification of children with cerebral palsy unable to maintain a normal nutritional state.' *Lancet*, **1**, 283–286.

Guo, S., Roche, A.F., Fomon, S.J., Nelson, S.E., Chumlea, W.C., Rogers, R.R., Baumgartner, R.N., Ziegler, E.E., Siervogel, R.M. (1991) 'Reference data on gains in weight and length during the first two years of life.' *Journal of Pediatrics*, **119**, 355–362.

Hamill, P.V.V., Drizd, T.A., Johnson, C.L., Reed, R.B., Roche, A.F., Moore, W.M. (1979) 'Physical growth: National Center for Health Statistics percentiles.' *American Journal of Clinical Nutrition*, **32**, 607–629.

Hammond, M.I., Lewis, M.N., Johnson, E.W. (1966) 'A nutritional study of cerebral palsied children.' *Journal of the American Dietetic Association*, **49**, 196–201.

Himes, J.H., Roche, A.F., Thissen, D., Moore, W.M. (1985) 'Parent-specific adjustments for evaluation of recumbent length and stature of children.' *Pediatrics*, **75**, 304–313.

Johnson, C.L., Fulwood, R., Abraham, S., Bryner, J.D. (1981) *Basic Data of Anthropometric Measurements and Angular Measurements of the Hip and Knee Joints for Selected Age Groups 1–74 Years of Age: United States 1971–75. Vital and Health Statistics Series 11, No. 219*. Hyattsville, MD: National Center for Health Statistics. (DHHS Publication No. (PHS) 81-1669.)

Johnson, R.K., Maeda, M. (1989) 'Establishing outpatient nutrition services for children with cerebral palsy.' *Journal of the American Dietetic Association*, **89**, 1504–1506.

Karle, I.P., Bleiler, R.E., Ohlson, M.A. (1961) 'Nutritional status of cerebral-palsied children.' *Journal of the American Dietetic Association*, **38**, 22–26.

Krick, J., Van Duyn, M.A.S. (1984) 'The relationship between oral-motor involvement and growth: a pilot study in a pediatric population with cerebral palsy.' *Journal of the American Dietetic Association*, **84**, 555–559.

—— Murphy, P.E., Markham, J.F.B., Shapiro, B.K. (1992) 'A proposed formula for calculating energy needs of children with cerebral palsy.' *Developmental Medicine and Child Neurology*, **34**, 481–487.

Leamy, C.M. (1953) 'A study of the food intake of a group of children with cerebral palsy in the Lakeville Sanatorium.' *American Journal of Public Health*, **43**, 1310–1317.

Lee, M.M.C. (1959) 'Thickening of the subcutaneous tissues in paralyzed limbs in chronic hemiplegia.' *Human Biology*, **31**, 187–193.

Lifshitz, F., Maclaren, N.K. (1973) 'Vitamin D-dependent rickets in institutionalized, mentally retarded children receiving long-term anticonvulsant therapy. I. A survey of 288 patients.' *Journal of Pediatrics*, **83**, 612–620.

Lohman, T.G., Roche, A.F., Martorell, R. (1988) *Anthropometric Standardization Reference Manual*. Champaign, IL: Human Kinetics Books.

Mimaki, T., Walson, P.D., Haussler, M.R. (1980) 'Anticonvulsant therapy and vitamin D metabolism: evidence for different mechanisms for phenytoin and phenobarbital.' *Pediatric Pharmacology*, **1**, 105–112.

Patrick, J., Boland, M., Stoski, D., Murray, G.E. (1986) 'Rapid correction of wasting in children with cerebral palsy.' *Developmental Medicine and Child Neurology*, **28**, 734–739.

Peeks, S., Lamb, M.W. (1951) 'Comments on the dietary practices of cerebral palsied children.' *Journal of the American Dietetic Association*, **27**, 870–876.

Phelps, W.M. (1951) 'Dietary requirements in cerebral palsy.' *Journal of the American Dietetic Association*, **27**, 869–870.

Pryor, H.B., Thelander, H.E. (1967) 'Growth deviations in handicapped children. An anthropometric study.' *Clinical Pediatrics*, **6**, 501–512.

Reilly, S., Skuse, D. (1992) 'Characteristics and management of feeding problems of young children with cerebral palsy.' *Developmental Medicine and Child Neurology*, **34**, 379–388.

Rempel, G.R., Colwell, S.O., Nelson, R.P. (1988) 'Growth in children with cerebral palsy fed via gastrostomy.' *Pediatrics*, **82**, 857–862.

Roche, A.F., Davila, G.H. (1974) 'Differences between recumbent length and stature within individuals.' *Growth*, **38**, 313–320.

—— Himes, J.H. (1980) 'Incremental growth charts.' *American Journal of Clinical Nutrition*, **33**, 2041–2052.

—— Mukherjee, D., Guo, S., Moore, W.M. (1987) 'Head circumference reference data: birth to 18 years.' *Pediatrics*, **79**, 706–712.

Ruby, D.O., Matheny, W.D. (1962) 'Comments on growth of cerebral palsied children.' *Journal of the American Dietetic Association*, **40**, 525–527.

Sanders, K.D., Cox, K., Cannon, R., Blanchard, D., Pitcher, J., Papathakis, P., Varella, L., Maughan, R. (1990) 'Growth response to enteral feeding by children with cerebral palsy.' *Journal of Parenteral and Enteral Nutrition*, **14**, 23–26.

Shapiro, B.K., Green, P., Krick, J., Allen, D., Capute, A.J. (1986) 'Growth of severely impaired children: neurological versus nutritional factors.' *Developmental Medicine and Child Neurology*, **28**, 729–733.

Slaughter, M.H., Lohman, T.G., Boileau, R.A., Horswill, C.A., Stillman, R.J., Van Loan, M.D., Bemben, D.A. (1988) 'Skinfold equations for estimation of body fatness in children and youth.' *Human Biology*, **60**, 709–723.

Snyder, R.G., Schneider, L.W., Owings, C.L., Reynolds, H.M., Golomb, D.H., Schork, M.A. (1977) *Anthropometry of Infants, Children and Youths to Age 18 for Product Safety Design*. Bethesda, MD: Consumer Product Safety Commission. (Report no. UM-HSRI-77-17.)

Spender, Q.W., Cronk, C.E., Stallings, V.A., Hediger, M.L. (1988) 'Fat distribution in children with cerebral palsy.' *Annals of Human Biology*, **15**, 191–196.

—— —— Charney, E.B., Stallings, V.A. (1989) 'Assessment of linear growth of children with cerebral palsy: use of alternative measures to height or length.' *Developmental Medicine and Child Neurology*, **31**, 206–214.

Stallings, V.A., Charney, E.B., Davies, J.C., Cronk, C.E. (1993*a*) 'Nutrition-related growth failure of children with quadriplegic cerebral palsy.' *Developmental Medicine and Child Neurology*, **35**, 126–138.

—— —— —— —— (1993*b*) 'Nutritional status and growth of children with diplegic or hemiplegic cerebral palsy.' *Developmental Medicine and Child Neurology*, **35**, 997–1006.

Sterling, H.M. (1960) 'Height and weight of children with cerebral palsy and acquired brain damage.' *Archives of Physical Medicine and Rehabilitation*, **41**, 131–135.

Tanner, J.M., Davies, P.S.W. (1985) 'Clinical longitudinal standards for height and height velocity for North American children.' *Journal of Pediatrics*, **107**, 317–329.

Thommessen, M., Heiberg, A., Kase, B.F., Larsen, S., Riis, G. (1991*a*) 'Feeding problems, height and weight in different groups of disabled children.' *Acta Paediatrica Scandinavica*, **80**, 527–533.

—— Kase, B.F., Riis, G., Heiberg, A. (1991*b*) 'The impact of feeding problems on growth and energy intake in children with cerebral palsy.' *European Journal of Clinical Health*, **45**, 479–487.

—— Riis, G., Kase, B.F., Larsen, S., Heiberg, A. (1991*c*) 'Energy and nutrient intakes of disabled children: do feeding problems make a difference?' *Journal of the American Dietetic Association*, **91**, 1522–1525.

Tobis, J.S., Saturen, P., Larios, G., Posniak, A.O. (1961) 'Study of growth patterns in cerebral palsy.' *Archives of Physical Medicine and Rehabilitation*, **42**, 475–481.

Tolman, K.G., Jubiz, W., Sannella, J.J., Madsen, J.A., Belsey, R.E., Goldsmith, R.S., Freston, J.W. (1975) 'Osteomalacia associated with anticonvulsant drug therapy in mentally retarded children.' *Pediatrics*, **56**, 45–51.

Wodarski, L.A. (1990) 'An interdisciplinary nutrition assessment and intervention protocol for children with disabilities.' *Journal of the American Dietetic Association*, **90**, 1563–1568.

WHO (1985) *Energy and Protein Requirements. Technical Report Series 724*. Geneva: World Health Organization.

8
DIAGNOSTIC IMAGING AND SPECIAL INVESTIGATIONS IN THE ASSESSMENT OF THE DISABLED CHILD

Eric Loveday

Diagnostic imaging forms an integral part of the assessment of feeding and nutritional problems in the disabled child. Special difficulties may be faced by the radiologist and radiographer in any department where such patients are seen infrequently, as the children are often unable to cooperate fully and specialized equipment may be required. Radiology can contribute to the nutritional work-up in many ways, but should always form part of the wider assessment in close consultation with all those involved in the patient's care. This chapter will focus on the evaluation of motor function in the upper gastrointestinal tract, with particular reference to swallowing, oesophageal motility and gastro-oesophageal reflux, and gastric emptying.

Assessing the disabled child in the radiology department
The multidisciplinary approach
Close cooperation between radiologists and other clinicians is necessary for imaging to be effective in any field, and nowhere is this more true than in the assessment of disabled children. Detailed clinical information, usually supplemented by discussion, is essential if the radiologist is to interpret imaging findings accurately.

Since the work pioneered by the Johns Hopkins Swallowing Center in Baltimore, those involved in the assessment of swallowing, and radiologists in particular, have become increasingly aware of the need for, and benefits of, a multidisciplinary approach. Not only does this lead to a more thorough assessment, it also encourages optimal communication among the professional staff and between staff and carers. The images can be reviewed, usually on videotape, discussed and explained, and repeated or further evaluated as necessary (Kramer 1989). If it is possible for the specialist speech and language therapist to be present during the radiological investigations this is clearly advantageous.

Adaptations and special equipment
The main problems of imaging disabled children are the lack of mobility, difficulty with positioning and limited cooperation. The standard fluoroscopy table is usually a hard flat surface, and uncomfortable even when the patient can lie flat. Some form of padding is therefore a basic requirement; radiolucent foam mattresses with washable covers are available in most departments. Many children will be best positioned seated, particularly if they suffer some form of flexion contracture, and adaptations can be made, for example using

commercially available child car restraints (with or without seat belts). In a few situations the child may be examined in an ordinary chair or in her wheelchair or buggy. This is particularly true of some studies of swallowing, but for examination of the lower oesophagus and stomach some form of reclining position is required. Even with specially designed equipment it may need all the ingenuity of the imaging team in order to achieve the accurate positioning required for swallowing studies. Examinations may be time consuming and on occasions frustrating, and patience is vital in order to achieve satisfactory results.

A fluoroscopy unit with overhead tube offers the best access and is usually the least frightening to the child patient, albeit at the expense of a slightly increased radiation dose to the handlers. This type of unit can often be operated by remote control however, and where possible the radiologist should choose this option rather than be directly involved in the positioning and feeding of the patient, as her cumulative radiation dose will be the highest of those among the team. Alternatively, standard undercouch equipment may be used in which the X-ray tube is beneath the couch and the image intensifier is above (and necessarily close to) the patient. This has the benefit of more effective radiation shielding, albeit with restricted access to the patient. A 'C-arm' mounting may be useful as this allows the angulation of the tube and image intensifier to be altered without the need to move the patient, although hard copy film for detailed examination may not then be available with some units.

Choice of recording format

This depends on the structure or function being examined. It is well established that a few 'spot films' are wholly insufficient for documentation of the complex and rapid events of swallowing. Frame rates of up to 10 frames per second are possible with 100 mm film recording devices that are fitted with many standard fluoroscopy outfits, but even this rate is generally regarded as inadequate for a detailed examination. Cineradiography, in which frame rates of 25 or even 50 frames per second can be achieved, for a while became the standard recording medium and for the first time allowed detailed frame by frame sequencing of the swallowing mechanism.

More recently however, with the advent of high resolution image intensifiers and high definition formats, video recording has become accepted as the medium of choice. It has the benefit of low cost and does not require particularly sophisticated equipment for playback (although a video recorder with frame-by-frame playback facility is required). On most modern fluoroscopy units the image can be edge-enhanced to improve definition prior to recording.

Choice of contrast medium

Barium sulphate suspension continues to be the mainstay of contrast examinations of the gastrointestinal tract in children. Its principal advantages are its high density, ability to coat mucosal surfaces, low toxicity and low cost. Its use is contraindicated where there is any suspicion of perforation, as it may cause a severe inflammatory reaction in the peritoneum or mediastinum. If aspirated it is fairly inert, although high-density formulations (rarely used in children) have been reported to cause an inflammatory reaction in the lungs of elderly patients (Gray *et al.* 1989). This is rare however, and in most cases of barium aspiration no clinical sequelae are seen, particularly if physiotherapy is arranged following the event. Thus in children who regularly aspirate small quantities of more irritant organic foodstuffs, the relative dangers of barium sulphate should not be exaggerated.

Water soluble contrast media contain iodine, which has a lower atomic number, and therefore a lower density, than barium and therefore requires a greater concentration for equivalent radiographic density. All water soluble contrast media are more expensive than barium formulations. The choice here lies between ionic, high osmolality compounds and the more expensive low osmolality, usually non-ionic equivalents. Ionic solutions such as Gastrografin® have a number of drawbacks: in particular they may cause significant fluid shift into the bowel lumen due to osmotic effect. Some may be absorbed causing further fluid imbalance. If aspirated into the lungs they may provoke severe pulmonary oedema, and their use is contraindicated therefore when there is any risk of aspiration, however slight—gastrograffin is far more toxic than barium in this situation. Moreover they may have a direct toxic effect on gastric mucosa if contact is prolonged.

Non-ionic and low osmolality water soluble contrast media on the other hand are much safer, having very low toxicity in virtually any body cavity or surface, and these are the agents of choice when perforation or aspiration are suspected. The high cost of these compounds prohibits their general use, but fortunately with the small quantities required for examining neonates, where they have their major application, this is less of a problem. Non-ionic media are also hyperosmolar, albeit to a lesser degree, and if diluted to plasma osmolality show insufficient radiographic density. Newer dimeric compounds under development may overcome this drawback, but none is likely to completely replace barium, which is physically inert and provides greater radiographic contrast and better mucosal detail.

The best results in any situation will be achieved by tailoring the choice of contrast medium to the individual patient. Above all, the most important factor in reducing contrast reactions is not so much the choice of agent, as the skill and care with which the examination is performed (Cohen 1987).

Assessment of swallowing

Clinical assessment may be inadequate in identifying pharyngeal dysmotility during swallowing, and diagnostic imaging techniques are usually required for complete assessment. Specialized tests of deglutition such as the barium swallow may allow broad categorization of swallowing abnormalities. It is important when employing these tests to remember that they are mainly descriptive and do not provide data regarding specific pathophysiological mechanisms.

Phases of swallowing

The normal swallow may be conveniently divided into oral, pharyngeal and oesophageal phases. In adults respiration is voluntarily suspended during the swallow, while in suckling infants the rhythmical coordination of sucking, swallowing and breathing is an additional important factor (Bu'Lock *et al.* 1990). These swallowing mechanisms are dealt with in detail elsewhere in this volume; suffice to say that the radiologist needs to be aware of the normal mechanisms, not only to aid interpretation but also to assist in tailoring the examination to the needs of the individual under study.

Imaging and swallowing function

BARIUM RADIOLOGY

The examination is usually begun by giving barium liquid suspension by mouth, by means of bottle, cup or syringe depending on the age and feeding ability of the patient being examined. [Cineradiographic studies of breast feeding have been described (Ardran *et al.* 1958) but cannot be justified in clinical practice in view of the known radiosensitivity of the human breast.] Cooperation may be facilitated by flavouring the mixture with fruit cordial. Infants may be examined supine at first or in a specially designed seat. Forcible restraint should be eschewed if at all possible, but the design of fluoroscopy units and radiation safety considerations preclude cradling of an infant in her mother's arms.

If a nasogastric tube is present it should be removed as it may interfere with normal swallowing and hinder image interpretation. It may be worth noting that if a child has been fed exclusively via a nasogastric tube from early infancy, it is likely that she will be markedly 'oro-aversive' and abreact strongly against anything introduced into her mouth. This will pose great difficulties for the radiologist.

It is usual to commence with a brief survey of the initial swallow from lips to stomach before proceeding with the detailed examination. This allows early detection of major tracheal aspiration—in which case the examination may have to be terminated—and of unsuspected anatomical abnormalities such as oesophageal stricture or vascular rings. The moving image is usually recorded on videotape, as described above, for later review and may be supplemented with 'hard copy' films as required. Screening times, as always, should be kept to a minimum, in order to keep radiation dose to patient and carers as low as possible.

Observation of the response of the patient to attempted feeding is an important and integral part of the examination, and episodes of choking or respiratory distress should similarly be observed and documented.

The oral and oropharyngeal phases of swallowing are best observed in the lateral projection. This allows visualization of tongue shape, position and movements, and coordination can be studied (Fig. 8.1). Nasal escape and laryngeal penetration by contrast medium are also best shown in the lateral view. Supplementary views may be made in the anteroposterior or oblique projections according to need, and these projections are favoured for examination of the distal oesophagus.

Following the liquid swallow, supplementary information may be gained by giving barium paste, or a biscuit coated with barium, to determine if foods with these consistencies are handled safely (Griggs *et al.* 1989).

The object of the imaging study is to optimize the management of the patient. On the simplest level, patients may be classified as 'safe' or 'unsafe' for oral feeding. More sophisticated analysis allows specific recommendations to be made with respect to the type and consistency of foods that can safely be given, and the optimum position for feeding the patient. This has been borne out in several published studies, although few data are currently

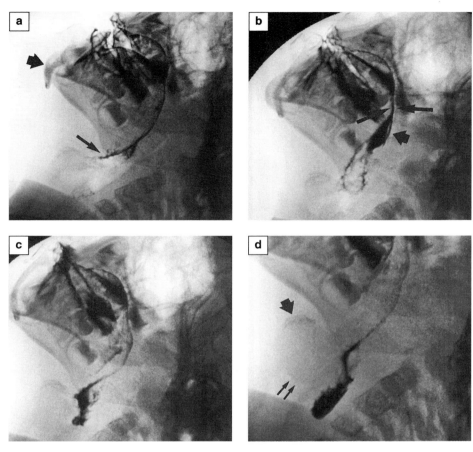

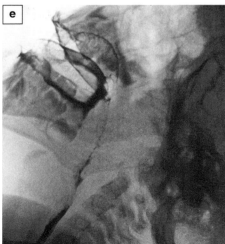

Fig. 8.1. Lateral view of barium swallow in 2-year-old child with cerebral palsy and a long history of feeding difficulties. The child is normally fed via a gastrostomy tube and is markedly oro-aversive. *(a)* Before swallow. Barium in the valleculae *(arrow)* should not be mistaken for laryngeal penetration, but may pose a risk of aspiration. Aversion and absent lip seal shown by barium on the chin *(short arrow)*. *(b–e)* The rapidity of the swallowing reflex is demonstrated by these images taken 0.125 s apart. *(b)* A small bolus *(short arrow)* is formed by the tongue compressing against the soft palate *(long arrows)*, but clearance of barium from the oral cavity is poor. *(c–e)* The swallow proceeds rapidly and safely. The position of the hyoid *(short arrow)* and undersurface of the vocal cords *(small arrows)* are easily appreciated in *(d)*. The patient has a normal swallowing reflex, but the abnormal oral phase and poor clearance of barium indicate a small risk of aspiration and choking.

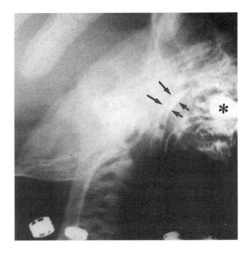

Fig. 8.2. Lateral barium contrast in an infant with choking episodes. The feeding teat *(asterisk)* is placed in the mouth. Poor palatal seal is shown by nasal escape of barium *(arrows)* over the upper surface of the soft palate *(short arrows)*. (Illustration courtesy of Dr Helen Carty.)

available on long term nutritional benefit (Griggs *et al.* 1989, Zerilli *et al.* 1990, Morton *et al.* 1993).

PALATAL FLUOROSCOPY

Direct observation of the palate with fluoroscopy can be used as a supplement to the swallow examination, although it more usually forms part of speech therapy assessment. Impaired palatal closure is manifested during the swallow as 'nasal escape' of liquid barium (Fig. 8.2). The palate may be observed during respiration and speech to look for symmetry and evidence of voluntary seal. The undersurface of the palate is usually coated with barium following the barium swallow and if fine detail is required the superior surface can be coated by dribbling a few drops of barium via a fine tube placed through the nares.

ULTRASOUND

Real-time ultrasound is a new technique in the assessment of swallowing. Modern scanners can achieve high resolution with rapid frame rates in excess of 25 frames per second which are thus comparable with videofluoroscopy and cineradiography. 'Cineloop' facilities on some scanners allow capture of an imaging sequence of up to four seconds for immediate frame by frame playback or replay at any desired speed; the examination can also be recorded on videotape for future analysis.

The major advantage of ultrasonography, particularly in the paediatric age group, is that it does not involve ionizing radiation; indeed at the dose rates used for diagnostic imaging it has no known hazards, and therefore not only can the examination be as long as is necessary but it may be repeated for follow-up. By its nature ultrasonography is physically flexible as the probe is mounted on a flexible lead, in contrast to the fluoroscopy unit where the patient needs to be positioned in relation to a large piece of fixed equipment.

For swallowing studies the probe is usually placed submentally where the soft tissues of the floor of the mouth provide an acoustic window through which the tongue, hyoid bone, larynx and to a lesser extent the posterior pharyngeal structures can be imaged. The scan-head used should be either a mechanical or phased array sector probe, or a curved linear array probe; these designs allow simultaneous visualization in the sagittal plane from the tongue anteriorly to the hyoid bone and larynx posteriorly. The presence of the probe in this position may potentially interfere with normal swallowing, although to some degree this can be overcome by selection of the best available probe design and the use of stand-off pads made of flexible gel.

Air and bone form barriers to high frequency sound transmission and this is a major impediment, as unless the tongue is kept apposed to the roof of the mouth the palate cannot be seen, and the examination is not suited therefore to the assessment of palatal movement or the detection of nasal escape. Any liquid such as milk or water can be used, and as for barium studies comparison can be made with the use of thicker pastes. In the author's experience it has not been possible to generate useful images with solid foods.

Imaging can take place in the coronal or sagittal planes, and because of flexible positioning it is simple to obtain a midline sagittal image. A fundamental difference compared with fluoroscopy is that the ultrasound image is cross-sectional. This has the advantage of avoiding confusion due to overlap of adjacent structures (as is seen with planar imaging), although on the other hand if the wrong scan plane is used information may be missed.

In the coronal plane the tongue musculature can be assessed for symmetry and resting activity. Nutritive and non-nutritive sucking movements can easily be assessed. During normal deglutitive action a pronounced 'V' shape is shown as the tongue accommodates and controls the bolus during propulsion to the back of the mouth. In the sagittal plane the oropharyngeal phase is shown as a smooth stripping wave from anterior to posterior, the magnitude of which depends on the size of the bolus (Kahrilas *et al.* 1993) and on the feeding skills of the patient under examination.

In children it is usually possible to follow the bolus as it passes from the posterior oropharynx through the cervical oesophagus. The major mechanism for airway protection is elevation of the hyoid, larynx and epiglottis as a unit, and this can easily be observed during the swallow. Systematic observation over several swallows will allow detection of abnormal movements of the tongue or hyoid, and coordination of the phases of swallowing can be assessed.

The larynx in children is sonolucent and by observing abduction of the cords during quiet inspiration it is possible to detect vocal cord palsies. Small amounts of liquid penetrating the larynx during the swallow will be missed, however, and ultrasound cannot replace the barium swallow in documenting aspiration.

As with the barium swallow, the examination of disabled children is hampered by the very small bolus sizes that can be normally accommodated, so that the elegant depictions of the swallowing action that are possible in normal individuals cannot be simulated. Nevertheless even the smallest bolus should trigger reflex activity of the swallowing mechanism, which may be impaired (or absent) on the one hand, or exaggerated and chaotic on the other.

A few studies have appeared in the literature concerning ultrasound and swallowing. Bu'Lock *et al.* (1990) were able to document the coordination between sucking, swallowing and respiration during a complete or nearly complete bottle feed in each of 14 normal infants. Smith *et al.* (1985) used ultrasound to demonstrate intra-oral activity during nutritive and non-nutritive sucking. Other authors (Sonies 1991, Stone 1991) have attested to the value of ultrasound in paediatric swallowing assessment. The role of ultrasonography remains to be defined but certainly would seem to merit further assessment.

Complementary techniques
OESOPHAGEAL MANOMETRY
Oesophageal manometry measures the pressure in the upper and lower oesophageal sphincters. It can be used to evaluate the level of co-ordination of propulsive waves in the oesophagus and has been helpful in further characterization of swallowing difficulty in adults. The technique has been used to assess the adequacy of sucking and pharyngeal contraction, and may be of particular value in distinguishing isolated cricopharyngeal achalasia and pharyngeal–cricopharyngeal incoordination, both of which may appear similar radiologically (Fisher *et al.* 1981).

Unfortunately the solid state probes, including the smaller ones for paediatric use, are currently rather stiff and thick. Crying secondary to the discomfort caused by the presence of the probe leads to huge swings in intrathoracic pressure which obliterate any subtle pressure changes due to oesophageal incoordination. The alternative is to sedate the patient—in this unphysiological situation one is not sure what is being measured. At the present time, therefore, the technology exists to measure oesophageal pressures and propulsive activity but the technique has not been demonstrated to be of value in assessment of oesophageal motility in disabled children.

EXETER DYSPHAGIA ASSESSMENT TECHNIQUE (EDAT)
The EDAT is a noninvasive portable apparatus designed to monitor the respiratory events accompanying swallowing. Its development followed the observation that complex but reproducible respiratory activity accompanies the swallowing reflex during normal swallowing in adults and children (Nishino *et al.* 1985). Studies using this equipment have shown that patients with neuromuscular dysphagia of primarily motor origin tend to preserve relatively normal respiratory activity, while those with sensory feedback deficiency show abnormal coordination of breathing and swallowing activity (Selley *et al.* 1990).

In a comparison of the EDAT with multidisciplinary assessment in 18 children, Parrott *et al.* (1992) found it a reliable diagnostic aid which assisted in the assessment of the degree of feeding impairment within each of the four feeding skills tested.

Oesophagus and gastro-oesophageal reflux
The identification of clinically significant gastro-oesophageal reflux (GOR) is an important part of the assessment of upper gastrointestinal function in disabled children. A certain amount of reflux may clearly be regarded as normal ('possetting' or 'spitting-up') in normal children up to the age of 1 year (Cleveland *et al.* 1983), and the challenge facing the clinician is the differentiation of 'clinically significant' reflux from 'normal' degrees of reflux. GOR is a treatable condition and hence it is important to confirm its presence and assess its severity.

**Grading of gastro-oesophageal reflux according to appearances on
barium examination***

Grade 1	Reflux into distal oesophagus only.
Grade 2	Reflux extending above carina but not into cervical oesophagus.
Grade 3	Reflux into cervical oesophagus.
Grade 4	Free persistent reflux into cervical oesophagus with a widely patent cardia (chalasia).
Grade 5	Reflux of barium with aspiration into the trachea or lungs.
Grade D	Delayed reflux; barium seen in oesophagus on delayed films.

*McCauley *et al.* (1978).

The mechanism underlying most cases of GOR is uncertain, but alterations in relative intra-abdominal and intrathoracic pressure may be important. Imaging studies have documented the presence of sliding hiatal hernias in some, as well as morphological changes such as a short intra-abdominal oesophagus, a reduction in the acute angle of the gastro-oesophageal junction, and an appearance of the gastro-oesophageal junction which has been coined the oesophageal 'beak' due to the appearance of barium in the gastric fundus 'pointing' into the distal oesophagus (Cleveland *et al.* 1983, Westra *et al.* 1990). In swallowing-impaired children abnormal oesophageal motility may also be important. The effect of posture has possibly been overstated, and therapeutic manoeuvres such as sleeping upright may in fact actually increase reflux.

Methods of investigation
The principal relevant investigation for confirming significant GOR is prolonged lower oesophageal pH monitoring. This is described in detail in Chapter 12. In current practice this is frequently supplemented by diagnostic imaging. Many centres will not rely on the results of a single investigation when considering surgical therapy, requiring two or more tests to be positive (Leonidas 1984, Johnson 1985, Meyers *et al.* 1985, Le Dosseur *et al.* 1989, Parker 1993).

BARIUM STUDIES
Barium radiology is the mainstay of imaging investigation of the upper gastrointestinal tract in children, and has been used in the routine investigation of GOR since the classification proposed by McCauley *et al.* (1978) (Table 8.1).

It should be borne in mind when employing this classification that it was designed for purely descriptive purposes, and that at the time no attempt was made to correlate the grade of reflux with the severity of symptoms or the presence of complications. It has nevertheless become the standard on which reporting is commonly based.

It is well known that there are severe limitations to the use of barium fluoroscopy in the assessment of GOR. In children it is particularly important to keep radiation dose to a minimum, and for this reason five minutes of intermittent fluoroscopy is usually regarded as the maximum acceptable limit. It is obvious, therefore, on the one hand that significant reflux occurring outside this time interval will be missed, and on the other that very brief episodes may also be missed in between pulses of fluoroscopy. Despite these limitations the technique is remarkably sensitive for the presence or absence of reflux; the major problem, in fact, appears to be lack of specificity. The predictive value of a positive result (*i.e.* the frequency of clinically significant GOR among those with evidence of reflux on fluoroscopic examination) has been placed as low as 54 per cent—little better than the toss of a coin (Arasu *et al.* 1980, Herbst 1981, Cleveland *et al.* 1983, Seibert *et al.* 1983, Leonidas 1984). Other studies have confirmed this lack of specificity (Johnson 1985, Meyers *et al.* 1985), and most would advocate more than one investigation before contemplating aggressive therapy.

These limitations notwithstanding, there can be no doubting the value of barium examination of the upper gastrointestinal tract. Although functional observations may be of limited value as described above, no single other investigation can provide as much important anatomical information. An important aspect in the investigation, of the vomiting infant in particular, involves ruling out a number of mainly obstructive lesions, from oesophageal strictures to duodenal obstructions and malrotation syndromes. Barium radiography, by providing detailed images of all the relevant structures, is ideally suited and versatile enough to identify most of these problems.

ULTRASOUND

Real time ultrasound is emerging as a new method for the imaging of GOR. Its major advantages from the imaging point of view are its non-invasiveness and the lack of radiation exposure, allowing the study to continue for as long as necessary. Further potential advantages are the ability to measure the length of the intra-abdominal oesophagus, by displaying the point at which it crosses the diaphragm, and to directly image the muscular wall and the angle of the gastro-oesophageal junction. A blunting of this angle, and a sign corresponding to the 'beak sign' of the barium study, may be seen and have been shown to correlate with severity of reflux (Westra *et al.* 1990).

Many studies (Naik *et al.* 1985, LeDosseur *et al.* 1989, Gomes and Menanteau 1991) have attested to the sensitivity of ultrasound in the detection of GOR. Opinions vary as to its utility in clinical practice: its proponents favour its high sensitivity (Naik and Moore 1984, Parker 1993) and safety, while its detractors point to the relatively time consuming nature of the study and difficulties which may be encountered with the uncooperative child (McAlister 1991).

With ultrasound it is normally possible to view the distal thoracic oesophagus as it passes behind the left atrium, and by angling the probe slightly, good views of the gastro-oesophageal junction can be achieved (Fig. 8.3). Gastric contents are usually echogenic due to the presence of air, and reflux is easily seen as an opening of the cardia with to-and-fro movement of the fluid, particularly in severe cases. The gastro-oesophageal junction is usually seen with the probe in the epigastrium using the left lobe of the liver as an acoustic window. In disabled children skeletal deformities may alter the relative positions of the organs, and

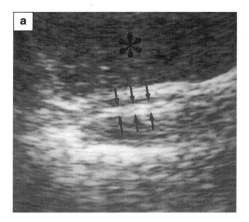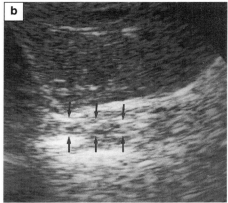

Fig. 8.3. Oblique longitudinal sonograms through the left lobe of the liver *(a—asterisk)* showing the intra-abdominal oesophagus posteriorly. *(a)* The closely opposed mucosal surfaces are visible as two parallel white stripes *(arrows)*. *(b)* A minor degree of gastro-oesophageal reflux causes separation of the mucosal layers *(arrows)*. In the 'real-time' examination the direction of movement of the refluxate is clearly evident.

frequently excessive amounts of bowel gas hinder good visualization, decreasing the success rate of ultrasound in this group. Surveillance may continue for 5–20 minutes, the length of time depending on local protocol, the compliance of the patient and the patience of the observer.

NUCLEAR MEDICINE

The scintigraphic technique involves giving the patient a liquid meal ('milk scan') by mouth or by tube. The meal contains a radiopharmaceutical, usually [99m]technetium labelled to sulphur colloid. Imaging of the stomach and oesophagus then takes place with a standard gamma camera placed under the patient. A typical examination will last for up to one hour with either continuous imaging or intermittent recordings at frequent regular intervals. Delayed images can be used to detect pulmonary aspiration of the radiopharmaceutical. Episodes of GOR can be documented visually or by plotting as a time–activity curve. The radiation burden to the patient is low, certainly less than the average barium meal.

The scintigraphic technique is a potentially attractive method for detecting GOR as surveillance of the tracer can continue for as long as necessary without any increase in the radiation dose to the patient. In theory, aspiration of stomach contents should be visible as activity in the bronchial tree. Functional information is combined with an anatomical display in the manner of a barium meal, but with the added possibility of quantitative assessment. Gastric emptying may also be assessed at the same time (Seibert *et al.* 1983; see below).

In a study comparing simultaneous one hour pH monitoring and scintigraphy in 49 patients, Seibert and coworkers found excellent correlation between episodes of reflux documented by the two techniques (Seibert *et al.* 1983). 47 patients also had 24 hour pH monitoring, and using this as their standard they found one hour scintigraphy had a sensitivity of 79 per cent and specificity of 93 per cent in detecting significant reflux. Barium examination performed on the same patients demonstrated a similarly high sensitivity but specificity using their criteria was very low at 21 per cent.

Scintigraphy is not without its problems, however. An optimal study with time–activity curves requires the patient to remain still for long periods of time. With good child handling skills, this can often be achieved in sleepy infants following a meal, but may be more problematical with the occasional anxious child. Lack of a standardized protocol, both in the method of the examination and in interpretation of results, has limited its value, and the technique has shown a disappointing lack of sensitivity in detecting pulmonary aspiration (Heyman 1985, Gordon 1986, Bowen 1988). Scintigraphy has so far not been applied to imaging of the upper gastrointestinal tract in children with cerebral palsy.

Choice of technique

The principal methods for investigating GOR in clinical practice are barium radiography, ultrasound, scintigraphy and extended lower oesophageal pH monitoring. The last mentioned is undoubtedly the most sensitive and specific method but is not without problems, being relatively invasive and relying on an acid stomach content in order to detect reflux. Any underlying anatomical abnormality may be missed, and the results of studies comparing the various techniques tend to indicate a complementary role (Leonidas 1984, Meyers *et al.* 1985, LeDosseur *et al.* 1989, Westra *et al.* 1990, Parker 1993). On the other hand, those investigations based on imaging (barium, ultrasound, scintigraphy) involve filling the stomach; it is precisely at this time that most reflux occurs in normal individuals so this may explain the lower specificity of these methods.

The barium examination, despite its lack of specificity, remains in widespread use, probably rightly so as no one technique can convey so much anatomical, and to a lesser degree functional, information regarding the oesophagus, stomach and proximal small bowel in such a short time. Ultrasonography is a promising technique and has the added advantage of being non-invasive; scintigraphy is also of proven value and can add quantitative information. Ultimately, however, the best results will usually involve a combination of tests, the choice of investigations depending on local expertise and interest.

Gastric emptying

The problems of GOR should not be considered in isolation since there is a large body of evidence suggesting that significant reflux is frequently accompanied by delayed gastric emptying (Hillemeier *et al.* 1983, Jolley *et al.* 1987, Papaila *et al.* 1989, LiVoti *et al.* 1992). The cause of this is unclear, and neither is it certain whether impaired gastric emptying predisposes to reflux in all cases, as would seem logical, or vice versa. For example, Hinder *et al.* (1989) showed that treating severe GOR by Nissen fundoplication resulted in normalization of gastric emptying times in patients with complications of reflux, while Maddern *et al.* (1985) showed significantly reduced rates of gastric emptying in patients with failed anti-reflux procedures. Gastric stasis may contribute to chronic undernutrition, as any patient whose stomach contains a large amount of residue is easily satiated following a relatively small meal.

Methods of assessment

Although barium studies, and to a lesser extent ultrasound, can detect gross degrees of gastric stasis and causes of anatomical gastric outlet obstruction, the mainstay of functional and quantitative assessment has been gamma scintigraphy. In a typical study the patient takes a meal comprising liquid or solid (or both) which has been labelled with a radioisotope, usually ^{99m}Tc. Activity over the stomach is monitored with a gamma camera over sequential time frames and plotted as a graph of activity versus time. The time taken for activity to reduce by one half may be measured as an index of gastric emptying, or alternatively the percentage reduction in activity at one hour.

A wide range of emptying times is seen in normal subjects, leading to difficulty in establishing a reference standard; this problem is compounded by the wide variety of techniques used in different centres. On the other hand, longitudinal studies of individual patients show a high degree of reproducibility making the technique valuable in assessing the response to treatment (Lawaetz and Dige-Petersen 1989, Maddern *et al.* 1991). This technique has yet to be applied to the study of gastric emptying in disabled children.

Such studies may be of value in disabled children who are being considered for gastrostomy feeding, a procedure known to worsen reflux; those with markedly prolonged emptying times may benefit from pyloroplasty in addition to an antireflux procedure. On the other hand pathologically reduced gastric emptying times ('dumping') have also been demonstrated in children (Lavine *et al.* 1988). Another useful application of the technique showed that whey-based formulas used for gastrostomy feeding were associated with shorter emptying times and fewer episodes of emesis than comparable casein-based formulas (Fried *et al.* 1992).

As indicated above, scintigraphic studies are the most commonly used in the investigation of gastric emptying but do carry the penalty of a small radiation dose. Techniques are under development which do not involve exposure to ionizing radiation. These include the use of a biosusceptometer to monitor the progress of test meals labelled with a harmless magnetic tracer (Miranda *et al.* 1992), and measurement of total gastric volumes and secretory rates during emptying, using magnetic resonance imaging (Schwizer *et al.* 1992). Epigastric impedance recording (Smith *et al.* 1993) is a technique that has been developed recently to study gastric emptying in children, and no doubt reports will soon appear detailing its usefulness when applied to disabled children. The role of these newer investigations remains to be defined.

REFERENCES

Arasu, T.S., Wyllie, R., Fitzgerald, J.F., Franken, E.A., Siddiqui, A.R., Lehman, G.A., Eigen, H., Grosfeld, J.L. (1980) 'Gastroesophageal reflux in infants and children—comparative accuracy of diagnostic methods.' *Journal of Pediatrics*, **96**, 798–803.

Ardran, G.M., Kemp, F.H., Lind, J. (1958) 'A cineradiographic study of breast feeding.' *British Journal of Radiology*, **31**, 156–162.

Bowen, A. (1988) 'The vomiting infant: recent advances and unsettled issues in imaging.' *Radiologic Clinics of North America*, **26**, 377–392.

Bu'Lock, F., Woolridge, M.W., Baum, J.D. (1990) 'Development of co-ordination of sucking, swallowing and breathing: ultrasound study of term and preterm infants.' *Developmental Medicine and Child Neurology*, **32**, 669–678.

Cleveland, R.H., Kushner, D.C., Schwartz, A.N. (1983) 'Gastroesophageal reflux in children: results of a standardized fluoroscopic approach.' *American Journal of Roentgenology*, **141**, 53–56.

Cohen, M.D. (1987) 'Choosing contrast media for the evaluation of the gastrointestinal tract of neonates and infants.' *Radiology*, **162**, 447–456.

Fisher, S.E., Painter, M., Milmoe, G. (1981) 'Swallowing disorders in infancy.' *Pediatric Clinics of North America*, **28**, 845–853.

Fried, M.D., Khoshoo, V., Secker, D.J., Gilday, D.L., Ash, J.M., Pencharz, P.B. (1992) 'Decrease in gastric emptying time and episodes of regurgitation in children with spastic quadriplegia fed a whey-based formula.' *Journal of Pediatrics*, **120**, 569–572.

Gomes, H., Menanteau, B. (1991) 'Gastro-esophageal reflux: comparative study between sonography and pH monitoring.' *Pediatric Radiology*, **21**, 168–174.

Gordon, I. (1986) 'Gastrointestinal scintigraphy in paediatrics.' *In:* Robinson, P.J.A. (Ed.) *Nuclear Gastroenterology.* Edinburgh, Churchill Livingstone, pp. 170–176.

Gray, C., Sivaloganathan, S., Simpkins, K.C. (1989) 'Aspiration of high-density barium contrast medium causing acute pulmonary inflammation—report of two fatal cases in elderly women with disordered swallowing.' *Clinical Radiology*, **40**, 397–400.

Griggs, C.A., Jones, P.M., Lee, R.E. (1989) 'Videofluoroscopic investigation of feeding disorders of children with multiple handicap.' *Developmental Medicine and Child Neurology*, **31**, 303–308.

Herbst, J.J. (1981) 'Gastroesophageal reflux.' *Journal of Pediatrics*, **98**, 859–870.

Heyman, S. (1985) 'Pediatric nuclear gastroenterology: evaluation of gastroesophageal reflux and gastrointestinal bleeding.' *In:* Freeman, L.M., Weissmann, H.S. (Eds.) *Nuclear Medicine Annual.* New York: Raven Press, pp. 133–165.

Hillemeier, A.C., Grill, B.B., McCallum, R., Gryboski, J. (1983) 'Esophageal and gastric motor abnormalities in gastroesophageal reflux during infancy.' *Gastroenterology*, **84**, 741–746.

Hinder, R.A., Stein, H.J., Bremner, C.G., DeMeester, T.R. (1989) 'Relationship of a satisfactory outcome to normalization of delayed gastric emptying after Nissen fundoplication.' *Annals of Surgery*, **210**, 458–464.

Johnson, D.G. (1985) 'Current thinking on the role of surgery in gastroesophageal reflux.' *Pediatric Clinics of North America*, **32**, 1165–1179.

Jolley, S.G., Leonard, J.C., Tunell, W.P. (1987) 'Gastric emptying in children with gastroesophageal reflux. I. An estimate of effective gastric emptying.' *Journal of Pediatric Surgery*, **22**, 923–926.

Kahrilas, P.J., Shezhang, L., Logemann, J.A., Ergun, G.A., Facchini, F. (1993) 'Deglutitive tongue action: volume accommodation and bolus propulsion.' *Gastroenterology*, **104**, 152–162.

Kramer, S.S. (1989) 'Radiologic examination of the swallowing impaired child.' *Dysphagia*, **3**, 117–125.

Lavine, J.E., Hattner, R.S., Heyman, M.B. (1988) 'Dumping in infancy diagnosed by radionuclide gastric emptying technique.' *Journal of Pediatric Gastroenterology and Nutrition*, **7**, 614–618.

Lawaetz, O., Dige-Petersen, H. (1989) 'Gastric emptying of liquid meals. A study in 88 normal persons.' *Annales Chirurgeriae et Gynaecologiae*, **78**, 267–276.

Le Dosseur, P., Beaudet, S., Oarda, M., Mouterde, W., Mallet, E., Eurin, D. (1989) 'Gastroesophageal reflux in infants: results of a standardized US study.' *Paper presented at the 26th Annual Congress of the European Society of Paediatric Radiology, Dublin, May 24–26, 1989.*

Leonidas, J.C. (1984) 'Gastroesophageal reflux in infants: role of the upper gastrointestinal series.' American Journal of *Roentgenology*, **143**, 1350–1351.

LiVoti, G., Tulone, V., Bruno, R., Cataliotti, F., Iacono, G., Cavataio, F., Balsamo, V. (1992) 'Ultrasonography and gastric emptying: evaluation in infants with gastroesophageal reflux.' *Journal of Pediatric Gastroenterology and Nutrition*, **14**, 397–399.

Maddern, G.J., Jamieson, G.G., Chatterton, B.E., Collins, P.J. (1985) 'Is there an association between failed antireflux procedures and delayed gastric emptying?' *Annals of Surgery*, **202**, 162–165.

—————— Myers, J.C., Collins, P.J. (1991) 'Effect of cisapride on delayed gastric emptying in gastro-oesophageal reflux disease.' *Gut*, **32**, 470–474.

McAlister, W.H. (1991) 'Gastrointestinal tract.' *In:* Siegel, M.J. (Ed.) *Pediatric Sonography.* New York: Raven Press, pp. 179–211.

McCauley, R.G.K., Darling, D.B., Leonidas, J.C., Schwartz, A.M. (1978) 'Gastroesophageal reflux in infants and children: a useful classification and reliable physiologic technique for its demonstration.' *American Journal of Roentgenology*, **130**, 47–50.

Meyers, W.F., Roberts, C.C., Johnson, D.G., Herbst, J.J. (1985) 'Value of tests for evaluation of gastroesophageal reflux in children.' *Journal of Pediatric Surgery*, **20**, 515–520.

Miranda, J.R., Baffa, O., de Oliveira, R.B., Matsuda, N.M. (1992) 'An AC biosusceptometer to study gastric emptying.' *Medical Physics*, **19**, 445–448.

Morton, R.E., Bonas, R., Fourie, B., Minford, J. (1993) 'Videofluoroscopy in the assessment of feeding disorders of children with neurological problems.' *Developmental Medicine and Child Neurology*, **35**, 388–395.

Naik, D.R., Moore, D.J. (1984) 'Ultrasound diagnosis of gastro-oesophageal reflux.' *Archives of Disease in Childhood*, **59**, 366–367.

—— Bolia, A., Moore, D.J. (1985) 'Comparison of barium swallow and ultrasound in diagnosis of gastro-oesophageal reflux in children.' *British Medical Journal*, **290**, 1943–1945.

Nishino, T., Yonezawa, T., Honda, Y. (1985) 'Effects of swallowing on the pattern of continuous respiration in human adults.' *American Review of Respiratory Disease*, **132**, 1219–1222.

Papaila, J.G., Wilmot, D., Grosfeld, J.L., Rescorla, F.J., West, K.W., Vane, D.W. (1989) 'Increased incidence of delayed gastric emptying in children with gastroesophageal reflux. A prospective evaluation.' *Archives of Surgery*, **124**, 933–936.

Parker, B.R. (1993) 'Disorders at the esophagogastric junction.' *In:* Silverman, F.N., Kuhn, J.P. (Eds.) *Caffey's Pediatric X-ray Diagnosis: an Integrated Imaging Approach.* St Louis: Mosby, pp. 1016–1026.

Parrott, L.C., Selley, W.G., Brooks, W.A., Lethbridge, P.C., Cole, J.J., Flack, F.C., Ellis, R.E., Tripp, J.H. (1992) 'Dysphagia in cerebral palsy: a comparative study of the Exeter Dysphagia Assessment Technique and a multidisciplinary assessment.' *Dysphagia*, **7**, 209–219.

Schwizer, W., Maecke, H., Fried, M. (1992) 'Measurement of gastric emptying by magnetic resonance imaging in humans.' *Gastroenterology*, **103**, 369–376.

Seibert, J.J., Byrne, W.J., Euler, A.R., Latture, T., Leach, M., Campbell, M. (1983) 'Gastroesophageal reflux—the acid test: scintigraphy or the pH probe?' *American Journal of Roentgenology*, **140**, 1087–1090.

Selley, W.G., Flack, F.C., Ellis, R.E., Brooks, W.A. (1990) 'The Exeter Dysphagia Assessment Technique.' *Dysphagia*, **4**, 227–235.

Smith, H.L., Hollins, G.W., Booth, I.W. (1993) 'Epigastric impedance recording for measuring gastric emptying in children: how useful is it?' *Journal of Pediatric Gastroenterology and Nutrition*, **17**, 201–206.

Smith, W.L., Erenberg, A., Nowak, A., Franken, E.A. (1985) 'Physiology of sucking in the normal term infant using real-time US.' *Radiology*, **156**, 379–381.

Sonies, B.C. (1991) 'Ultrasound imaging and swallowing.' *In:* Jones, B., Donner, M.W. (Eds.) *Normal and Abnormal Swallowing.* New York: Springer-Verlag, pp. 109–117.

Stone, M. (1991) 'Imaging the tongue and vocal tract.' *British Journal of Disorders of Communication*, **26**, 11–23.

Westra, S.J., Wolf, B.H.M., Staalman, C.R. (1990) 'Ultrasound diagnosis of gastroesophageal reflux and hiatal hernia in infants and young children.' *Journal of Clinical Ultrasound*, **18**, 477–485.

Zerilli, K.S., Stefans, V.A., DiPietro, M.A. (1990) ' Protocol for the use of videofluoroscopy in pediatric swallowing dysfunction.' *American Journal of Occupational Therapy*, **44**, 441–446.

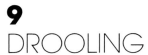

9
DROOLING

Peter A. Blasco

Drooling, or sialorrhea, is the unintentional loss of saliva and other oral contents from the mouth. It is a normal phenomenon of infancy that subsides in early childhood, usually by 15–18 months of age. Occasional drooling may persist in the neurologically intact child throughout the preschool years, but drooling during wakefulness beyond 3 or 4 years of age is considered abnormal (Crysdale 1989). Persistence into school age leads to social isolation, and the problem can be both practically and socially devastating in adolescence and adulthood (Creech 1991, Prentice 1991, Williams 1991). Drooling children frequently have chronically irritated, macerated facial skin, and in cool months the dampness from saliva is chilly. Dehydration can even become a recurrent problem as a consequence of chronic fluid and nutrient loss (Bailey and Wadsworth 1985, Blasco *et al.* 1991). Books and papers become untidy or damaged in school or at work, and electronic devices may malfunction. The ability of motor-impaired individuals to access new and sophisticated electronic technology that can offer them more opportunity to communicate and more independence is severely compromised by uncontrolled sialorrhea. Inability to control drooling in the face of peer pressure to do so can result in substantial loss of self-esteem. Besides being unsightly, concerns related to hygiene and disagreeable odor alienate people. Speech spray from individuals with wet mouths is unpleasant, and cough or sneeze can be a social catastrophe. For those naive to the problems of the developmentally disabled, it requires a conscious, learned effort to approach the drooler, enter into conversation, or make physical contact.

Problem drooling affects a small number of individuals in our society, mostly those with neurologic dysfunction in the form of motor deficits (*e.g.* cerebral palsy, peripheral neuromuscular disease, facial paralysis) or severe mental retardation. Cerebral palsy (CP) is diagnosed in 0.2–0.5 per cent of all children (Lipkin 1991), and an additional 0.2–0.7 per cent of the general population is retarded to a severe or profound degree. Although prevalence data for drooling have not been systematically gathered and reported, it is repeatedly estimated that 10 per cent of children with CP have drooling problems significant enough to interfere with daily social and practical functions (Ekedahl *et al.* 1974, Sochaniwskyj 1982, Blasco *et al.* 1992). An unknown number of retarded individuals are further handicapped by their drooling. A much smaller population of individuals exists who have lost the structural integrity of the jaw and/or lips as a result of trauma or oropharyngeal tumors with resultant chronic drooling. In itself, drooling affects the general well-being of the individual, and secondarily it may present problems for caregivers. Therefore its early recognition and specific treatment is essential to the overall intervention plan of the multidisciplinary team. The goal is to promote a better quality of life and to improve social interactions.

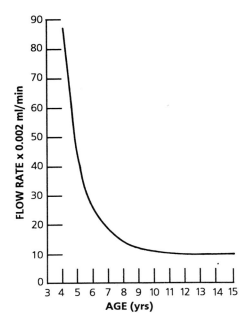

Fig. 9.1. Age *vs* rate of flow (× 0.002 ml/min) of unstimulated parotid saliva. (Reproduced by permission from Lourie 1943.)

From a research perspective, studies are needed to better define the populations involved and to determine prevalence and severity of drooling in a representative sample of people with CP. A study of successful adults in whom drooling persists has been proposed to address how they learn to cope with the problem and how successful their coping strategies are.

Salivary physiology

Saliva serves a number of very important functions. It aids in protecting the teeth from decay and the gingival tissues from inflammation and periodontal disease. It keeps the oral mucosa comfortably moist and acts as a lubricant for promoting swallowing and as a solvent for facilitating taste. It provides a cleansing and antibacterial action in the mouth cutting down on breath odor. Lastly, it promotes digestion through various enzymes, pH modulation and other factors (Myer 1989, Kaplan and Baum 1993).

Saliva production varies, averaging 0.5–1.5 litres daily in the adult. Flow rate diminishes with age (Fig. 9.1), and there is extensive person-to-person variation depending on environmental stimuli and conditions (Lourie 1943, Schneyer and Levin 1954). This becomes a major issue in measurement and in diagnostic evaluation, especially among younger children. The composition and viscosity of saliva produced by the different glands varies (Schneyer and Levin 1954). The submandibular and sublingual glands produce a high viscosity fluid which accounts for 70 per cent of the resting saliva. The more watery parotid secretions account for 20–25 per cent, and the rest is supplied by the minor palatal and mucosal glands (Dawes 1978).

93

Spectrum of oral-motor dysfunction

Problem drooling spans a continuum of severity. *Mild* droolers spill saliva onto their lips but not beyond the vermilion border. *Moderate* drooling reaches the chin, and *severe* drooling is characterized by dripping onto clothing. Those with the greatest problem experience *profuse* drooling: books, papers, equipment and every other possession in proximity to the face gets soaked (Blasco and Allaire 1992).

The standard concept of drooling refers to visible anterior (or labial) spill. However, individuals with oral-motor dysfunction also have oral retention in sublingual and buccal pools, pharyngeal retention, and a clinically more serious posterior spill through the faucial isthmus. The pooling of saliva, at times mixed with food, may be the mechanism of malodor. The term 'posterior drooling' has been applied to the situation in which oral secretions are not lost externally but rather pool in the hypopharynx where they should normally stimulate a swallow reflex (Blasco and Allaire 1992). In the absence of adequate swallowing they spill over into the pharynx producing congested breathing, coughing and gagging, vomiting, and at times aspiration into the trachea. Though severe oral-motor dysfunction is a factor in posterior drooling, there is likely a significant pharyngeal sensory deficit or a central disruption of the sensorimotor connection, interfering with reflex swallowing (Ekedahl *et al.* 1974, Blasco and Allaire 1992). Burgmayer and Jung (1983) suggested that insufficient sensory appreciation of external salivary loss was the main cause of drooling in children with mental retardation and CP. One group of investigators found evidence for intra-oral sensory dysfunction in children and young adults with CP and sialorrhea (Weiss-Lambrou *et al.* 1988).

Viewed in this broader context, anterior drooling (sialorrhea) represents one element on a continuum of oral performance impairments which include speech (articulation) problems, feeding and swallowing difficulty, upper respiratory congestion, and even aspiration. Indeed, severe drooling without associated speech impairment is virtually unheard of, while drooling associated with normal speech will almost always be mild and should probably never be treated surgically (Brody 1977).

The term sialorrhea implies excessive secretion of saliva, though most assert that saliva is not over-produced in children who drool but that inadequate swallowing and lip closure are the problems (Goode and Smith 1970, Koheil *et al.* 1987, Myer 1989). Sochaniwskyj *et al.* (1986) and Lespargot *et al.* (1993) have provided support for this clinical observation in their comparison of normal subjects and children with CP. They studied drinking tasks and found that children with CP who drooled had more trouble with lip closure and swallowing mechanics than unimpaired children or children with CP who did not drool. Lashley (1917) reported an increased rate of salivation in subjects with adult-onset hemiplegia. Collecting from individual parotid glands, he found markedly increased basal secretion rates in three of nine subjects and unpredictable responses to stimuli (exaggerated rises or decreases in secretion). Secretion rate from the gland on the hemiparetic side was consistently faster, but there was little correlation between rate of secretion and clinical sialorrhea. Lourie (1943) reported the same finding of hypersecretion in a few subjects that he studied. Of course, these two phenomena are not incompatible; that is, some children with CP may have both increased salivation and decreased or ineffective swallowing.

Treatment

Many modalities—various therapies, medications to dry secretions, surgery to alter or eliminate gland function, even radiation—have been proposed, often in combination, to treat drooling. No one option is universally successful, and many treatments have potential complications. Adults with CP and parents of disabled children typically assert fears about surgery, scepticism about drugs, and disappointment or frustration with positioning and behavioral interventions (Blasco and Allaire 1992). The literature on these treatments is often conflicting in terms of the conclusions reached and is rarely helpful in determining the best approach for the individual patient.

All existing research studies demonstrate a major weakness in the methodology used to quantify drool volume. This lack of an effective measurement system hinders the interpretation of individual studies and their comparison to each other.

The literature currently provides no comparisons between different interventions (surgery *vs* medication, medication *vs* behavioral treatment, etc.). In order to achieve such comparisons, collaboration among different centers and a uniform database to provide systematic information about the characteristics of each patient will be necessary (Blasco and Allaire 1992).

Hands-on therapy and behavioral treatments

Since positional and oral functional problems predispose to drooling, it follows that treatments to improve body position and posture along with specific oral-motor therapy have an important place in the management of drooling. Occupational, physical and speech/language therapists employ handling techniques and the use of assistive equipment to enhance head control, normalize muscle tone and stabilize body position. These aspects of treatment are addressed in Chapter 11. The intent is to promote jaw stability, to elicit mouth and lip closure, to decrease tongue thrust and to facilitate swallowing. Most reports of oral-motor therapy represent only one- or two-subject studies or are anecdotal case descriptions. In a small study (10 subjects) designed to control for this type of intervention, Boullard (1984) found little difference between treated and untreated groups, though certain individuals did clearly improve with therapy. Harris and Dignam (1980) used an external device, a chin cup, plus therapy. They compared a group of droolers treated with chin cups plus oral musculature training against a group managed with the training program alone and a group of untreated controls. Both treatment groups improved but benefits were greater for those receiving combined treatment. In general there is a striking paucity of clinical research to document the effectiveness of neurodevelopmental therapies in the area of oral-motor dysfunction and, specifically, drooling control (Ottenbacher *et al.* 1983). Even less can be said about the utility of oral appliances combined with therapy (Haberfellner and Rossiwall 1977, Shavell 1977, Nelson *et al.* 1981, Limbrock *et al.* 1990).

Behavior modification programs to promote awareness of salivary escape and to encourage regular swallowing have been advocated. Although most of the published behavior modification studies also suffer from the problem of small sample size, rigorous single-subject design methodology has often been employed (Garber 1971, Richman and Kozlowski 1977, Drabman *et al.* 1979, Thorbecke and Jackson 1982, Trott and Maechtlen 1986, Dunn *et al.*

1987). Dunn *et al.* (1987) used a multiple baseline design across clinical and educational settings with an adolescent male. While external cues (verbal prompts) were helpful, generalization to other settings was dependent on periodic re-initiation of treatment. This study emphasized the internal control learned by the subject. Thorbecke and Jackson (1982) had similar success using praise, overcorrection, habit reversal, criticism and self-instruction with an adolescent with mental retardation and mild CP.

Koheil *et al.* (1987) meticulously studied the efficacy of EMG biofeedback in 12 children with CP. Though most of the subjects were nonverbal, none were severely retarded. The authors quantified rate of drooling by using Sochaniwskyj's (1982) chin cup and by counting frequency of swallowing. Oral-motor control was trained using biofeedback from mouth (orbicularis oris) and neck (infrahyoid) muscles used in swallowing. Swallowing frequency was then increased by training with a timed auditory cue. The rate of drooling decreased significantly in conjunction with this cued behavior modification technique. Drooling remained decreased up to one month after completion of the study in nine of the 12 subjects. Although there was a slight initial increase in swallowing rates, it was not significant, leading the authors to conclude that swallowing became more proficient rather than more frequent.

Research into the mechanics of swallowing dysfunction in CP populations is gaining momentum (Sochaniwskyj *et al.* 1986, Bosma *et al.* 1990, Casas *et al.* 1990, Vice *et al.* 1990, Lespargot *et al.* 1993, Casas *et al.* 1994). Current studies of swallowing using non-invasive techniques like ultrasound (Smith *et al.* 1985, Bosma *et al.* 1990, Casas *et al.* 1990) and cervical auscultation (Vice *et al.* 1990) should be coupled with clinical information about both anterior and posterior drooling.

Without using special equipment for biofeedback, Rapp (1980) also trained a group of children with CP and mental retardation to swallow more frequently in response to an auditory cue. Rapp pointed out that success was greater in children with higher mental ages. However, Jones (1982) was unable to duplicate the success of this project. Subjects were tested for drool control under two conditions: when not involved in a task and when concentrating on a demanding task. Group results showed no significant decrease in either situation after 7–8 weeks of intervention, but there was considerable intra-subject variability. Parents, teachers, and patients themselves note that as long as an individual concentrates on a behavioral intervention drooling is reduced, but as soon as she loses concentration or focuses on another task the improvements are erased (Creech 1991, Williams 1991). Lourie (1943), studying the basic physiology of salivary secretion, found that most normal subjects decreased their rates with concentration except for some children who would increase. In contrast, all mentally retarded subjects he studied increased salivary secretion with concentration. Jones emphasized the need for careful description of the type and degree of motor impairment and a quantitative measure of mental capacity for each subject.

In these behavioral and oral-motor therapy studies there is generally a paucity of evaluation of labial motor performance. Drooling is never completely eliminated, only decreased to some variable degree. Carry-over to the second baseline condition is typically incomplete, with at times major losses of the initial benefits. The problem of generalization to other settings is inconsistently addressed. On the positive side, little in the way of specialized skill is needed for this approach. Bronwen Jones (1993) has put together a concise, practical outline of basic behavioral interventions. In the same book (Johnson and Scott 1993), there is also an excellent guide to compensatory management strategies (clothing, odor control, etc.). Further research into odor management through the use of chemicals applied to clothing to reduce odors and through information about specific foods that lead to disagreeable salivary odors is worth pursuing.

Pharmacologic approach

Salivation is mediated through the autonomic nervous system primarily by way of the cholinergic system's muscarinic receptor sites. Blockade of these receptors inhibits nervous stimulation to the salivary glands thereby reducing drooling. Anticholinergic drugs have widespread effects manifested at all end organs that are governed by muscarinic stimulation, and there is little selectivity in terms of blocking transmission at only the desired site. Because of their effects on oral and airway secretions, anticholinergic drugs have long been favored as pre-anesthetic agents, and atropine, the classic antimuscarinic agent, has the added beneficial effect of dilating the bronchi and bronchioles through smooth muscle relaxation. Variations in the structure of natural and synthetic compounds result in somewhat different quantitative actions at different organs (Blasco and Allaire 1992). For example, central stimulation consisting of restlessness, irritability and even delirium are side-effects of atropine, whereas mild sedation is more commonly produced by scopolamine. Known physiologic effects of the administration of anticholinergic agents parallel the side-effects often reported in therapeutic efficacy studies (Table 9.1).

A large number of drugs have been tried in an effort to diminish drooling. Antihistamines and more specific anticholinergic agents are the most commonly employed. The general clinical wisdom, based on anecdotal experience, has been to dismiss these agents (Arnold and Gross 1977, Brody 1977, Guerin 1979, Bailey and Wadsworth 1985, Crysdale 1989). Scopolamine delivered by a skin patch has generated a great deal of clinical interest because of its easy use (Talmi *et al.* 1990, Siegel and Klingbeil 1991, Lewis *et al.* 1994). Lewis *et al.* (1994) found good efficacy and little in the way of side-effects in 10 severely impaired children using the patch. However, it may be more toxic than generally appreciated (Wilkinson 1987, Ziskind 1988). Benztropine ('Cogentin'), a synthetic antimuscarinic, was studied in a placebo-controlled, double-blind fashion by Camp-Bruno *et al.* (1989). 20 individuals (age range 4–44 years), 19 of whom had CP, were treated. Three additional subjects were eliminated from the study because of severe anticholinergic side-effects, and four additional subjects were excluded because of recurrent acute illnesses. All subjects experienced severe drooling and more than half were severely to profoundly retarded. Except for the patients eliminated, side-effects were minimal and could be reduced with dosage adjustments. Based on a drooling scale rated by teachers, 85 per cent of the subjects studied responded to the drug, but 35 per cent also responded to placebo. Among the responders, drooling was not abolished but was reduced by 40–50 per cent, something that pleased teachers. Though long term efficacy was not specifically addressed, slightly more than 50 per cent of those treated stayed on medication and continued to benefit from it after the study was completed. In a similar study, Reddihough *et al.* (1990) employed benzhexol ('Artane') to treat severe

TABLE 9.1
Effects of muscarinic blockade

CNS: stimulation/depression

Eyes: pupillary dilation (photophobia) and cycloplegia (blurred vision); decreased tearing

Ear, nose and throat: decreased secretion (dry nose), decreased vestibular response

Salivary glands: decreased secretion (xerostomia)

Bronchi: small airway dilation

Heart: tachycardia

Stomach and intestines: decreased secretions; decreased motility (constipation)

Bladder: decreased detrusor muscle tone (diminished/delayed emptying)

Skin: decreased sweating (increased temperature, flushing)

Muscle: decreased tone, decreased adventitious movement

---

drooling in 20 children with CP (age range 3–12 years). All had failed to respond to behavioral programs. Baseline drooling rates showed great inter- and often intra-subject variability. Responses also varied tremendously from little or none in eight children to virtually complete cessation of drooling in three. Three families reported mild drug side-effects, and some continued the drug for 1–2 years after completion of the study because of the benefits. As with behavioral treatments, drug studies rarely demonstrate more than partial improvement in subjects who respond.

Glycopyrrolate ('Robinul') is a quaternary ammonium antimuscarinic compound structurally related to atropine. This drug has become popular with anesthetists as a pre-anesthetic agent and with pulmonologists for controlling secretions in younger children who have tracheostomies and have difficulty managing their secretions. Its advantages are that it has a long action and does not cross the blood–brain barrier. Hence central side-effects are greatly diminished, an advantage over benztropine which often produces sedation or, less commonly, dysphoria and restlessness. In my experience, glycopyrrolate has been moderately effective and relatively benign (Blasco and Stansbury 1996). Dosage guidelines for children are poorly delineated. Our patients have ranged in age from 4 years to young adulthood and have received dosages ranging from 0.04–0.4 mg/kg/day divided into two to four doses with a maximum total daily dose of 8 mg.

No one drug is perfectly selective, so use of antimuscarinics of necessity carries a price in terms of side-effects. A characteristic of these agents is their tendency to be most effective in situations where excessive parasympathetic stimulation is at the root of the problem (Weiner 1980). In other words, pharmacotherapy is most likely to be effective where salivation is excessive, a situation believed to be uncommon in the CP population. This may not, however, be a valid assumption in the light of the work of Lashley (1917) and Lourie (1943) cited previously. Though there exists a general pessimism about pharmacologic management, recent studies (Camp-Bruno *et al.* 1989, Reddihough *et al.* 1990, Dworkin and Nadal 1991, Lewis *et al.* 1994) suggest somewhat greater optimism. If there is a subgroup of patients in which the production of secretions is, in fact, quantitatively increased, this might be the group most suitable for pharmacologic management.

Surgical approaches
Ablation of one or more salivary glands decreases the quantity of saliva and alters its viscosity. Bilateral parotid gland excision, for example, leaves a thicker, mucoid saliva secreted by the submaxillary glands (the paired submandibular and sublingual glands) and no longer diluted by the more serous fluid supplied by the parotids. Removing all salivary flow is undesirable because of the adverse effects of xerostomia on oral and pharyngeal comfort, on dental health, and on the ability to masticate and swallow food. In persons with sialorrhea that is not based on neurologic dysfunction, surgical procedures which remove walls of soft tissue or scar that dam up salivary pools will directly improve swallowing mechanics. For some, biologic or prosthetic channels have been constructed that rely on gravity to drain saliva from pools formed in the anterior oral cavity. These conduits bypass the larynx and release the saliva at a lower level in the cervical oesophagus. In other situations, reconstruction of congenital or acquired deformities of the tongue or jaw may restore swallowing mechanics.

Radiation to the parotid and submandibular glands was formerly advocated as a method to suppress salivary secretion but has been appropriately criticized and abandoned, at least in the pediatric population, because of the long term hazards of growth arrest and radiation injury (Goode and Smith 1970, Arnold and Gross 1977, Brody 1977, Fear *et al.* 1988). Even small doses of radiation in children are known to produce skin and thyroid cancers, leukemia, and growth arrest with facial asymmetry (Martin *et al.* 1970, Vaughan 1971, Davis *et al.* 1989, US Health and Human Services 1989).

Otolaryngologists generally favour interrupting the parasympathetic nerve supply to the salivary glands. This accomplishes in a highly selective fashion what pharmacologic therapy cannot do. The submaxillary glands receive innervation from the submandibular ganglion by way of preganglionic fibres in the chorda tympani, a branch of the facial nerve (cranial nerve VII) (Fig. 9.2). Parotid innervation arrives from the brainstem via cranial nerve IX travelling through Jacobson's nerve, the tympanic plexus and the otic ganglion (Michel *et al.* 1977, Myer 1989). Surgical neurectomy must be complete in order to abolish both submaxillary and parotid stimulation (Goode and Smith 1970, Michel *et al.* 1977, Mullins *et al.* 1979). Loss of taste to the anterior aspect of the tongue is often mentioned (Arnold and Gross 1977, Brody 1977, Wilkie and Brody 1977, Mullins *et al.* 1979, Bailey and Wadsworth 1985, Sellars 1985, Shott *et al.* 1989), but among the surgeons there is no agreement as to its extent or the significance to the patient. Data on any functional deficit actually experienced by the persons involved are lacking, though Charles Gross (1990), who has the most extensive experience with neurectomy, denies that altered taste ever occurs. Toremalm and Bjerre (1976) and Michel *et al.* (1977) report no ill effects on weight or on feeding capability in their studies. In summary, the early response to this type of surgery is generally quite good, but over time the benefits become much less consistent.

Some plastic surgeons and oral surgeons favor procedures on the salivary glands or

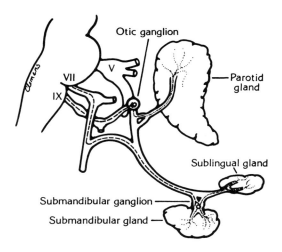

Fig. 9.2. Parasympathetic innervation of the salivary glands. (Reproduced by permission from Myer 1989.)

Otic ganglion

V

VII

IX

Parotid gland

Sublingual gland

Submandibular ganglion

Submandibular gland

their ducts. Methods include extirpation of the parotid and/or submandibular and/or sublingual glands, ligating or relocating the parotid ducts, and relocating the submandibular ducts. A combined approach pioneered by Wilkie and Brody (1977) and now referred to as the 'Wilkie procedure' involves removal of the submandibular glands and repositioning of the parotid ducts to a more posterior location in the area of the tonsillar fossae (Guerin 1979, Rosen *et al.* 1990). Parotid duct ligation, rather than repositioning, is vigorously advocated by others (Dundas and Peterson 1979, Brown *et al.* 1985, Brundage and Moore 1989). Faggella and Osborn (1983) concluded that *both* (ligation on one side and repositioning on the other) were optimum. Crysdale and White (1989), who favor relocation of the submandibular ducts and excision of the small sublingual glands, reported great success in 194 patients seen in a referral clinic. They believe the key to success with duct rerouting procedures may actually be due to an increased pharyngeal stimulus to swallow. If this is true, surgical relocation of salivary flow may represent a more direct treatment of the fundamental swallowing problem in drooling than first appears. However, using nuclear scintigraphy, Crysdale (unpublished data) and others (Pogrel 1987, Hotaling *et al.* 1992) have observed complete or partial cessation of gland function following rerouting. Presumably, this is based on inadvertent duct kinking or other obstruction with resultant glandular fibrosis and atrophy (as occurs with simple duct ligation).

Many clinicians point out that nasopharyngeal obstruction causes mouth-open posture and thereby is a strong promoter of drooling. They cite several 'cures' following tonsillectomy and adenoidectomy. The most common complication of surgery on the floor of the mouth is ranula formation. These submucosal saliva-containing cysts can expand to uncomfortable size, often require surgical treatment, and may recur (Guerin 1979, Bailey and Wadsworth 1985, Crysdale and White 1989). Arnrup and Crossner (1990) have raised concern about an increase in dental caries, localized to the lower incisors and canines, in patients undergoing submandibular gland procedures. In general, each procedure has its own set of complications and/or undesirable side-effects such as respiratory compromise, infection, cyst or hematoma formation, xerostomia, pain, swelling and visible scarring. Burton (1991) has thoroughly reviewed the history of these many procedures, concluding that "each . . . has its devotees and detractors". Because of each surgeon's enthusiasm, the surgical literature is extremely difficult to evaluate. As seen in other treatment studies, measurement techniques, outcome measures and long term follow-up are areas of weakness in most of these surgical reports. Surgical approaches need to be studied in a comparative manner in an effort to settle the controversy over neurectomy *vs* gland procedures.

While most published surgical experience is very positive, a number of parents have reported that their children were worse-off following surgery (see Blasco *et al.* 1991). Stevenson *et al.* (1994) describe an adolescent with CP who went from safe functional oral feeding to progressive dysphagia, weight loss and aspiration pneumonia following duct rerouting. This adverse experience may be under-reported or at least underemphasized in the surgical literature. At the Hugh MacMillan Rehabilitation Centre in Toronto, all surgical cases have been followed longitudinally and, of over 200 patients operated on with a variety of surgeries, none were worse after the procedure. The non-successes were all "no change" (Crysdale 1989). Clearly the obvious benefits that follow surgical control of drooling must be balanced in each case against the potential drawbacks. Unfortunately there does not appear to be a method for prospectively identifying those at most risk of having an adverse outcome from surgery. Brody (1977) and Edgerton (personal communication, 1991) have both alluded to greater difficulties in children with severe athetosis, just as encountered in the case reported by Stevenson *et al.* (1994). Indeed, criteria for selecting surgical candidates are rarely addressed beyond the general indicators for treating sialorrhea (Blasco 1992).

Crysdale and White (1989) strongly advocate an interdisciplinary team assessment and hierarchical treatment plan advancing to surgery when other interventions have proved unsatisfactory. Their team at the Hugh MacMillan Centre consists of an otolaryngologist, a pediatric dentist and a speech pathologist. Treatment recommendations are developed through a group decision-making process and are based on clinical evaluation of the type and severity of drooling and associated structural or neurodevelopmental problems. The parents and patients are included in developing a step-wise plan leading to either no immediate treatment, intervention with hands-on therapy or equipment, biofeedback, pharmacotherapy, or surgery. Of over 500 persons evaluated, about 70 per cent have come to surgery (Crysdale 1989). However, this is a highly selected referral population of severe droolers, most of whom are mentally retarded as well as motor impaired and almost all of whom have received extensive previous interventions.

In conclusion, based on current experience there would appear to be five factors potentially operative in the development of pathological drooling: (1) integrity of the oral structures, especially lips, tongue and jaw; (2) oropharyngeal motor function; (3) orofacial sensory perception and feedback; (4) rate of saliva secretion; and (5) cognitive appreciation of salivary spill. Although precise determination and clear separation of each factor is not always possible, treatment can to some extent be tailored to the evaluation of dysfunction in each area. For example, in profoundly retarded individuals, behavioral treatment programs will tend to be less effective and may require frequent re-establishment. If substantial aspiration and recurrent bouts of pneumonia were well-documented, duct rerouting might diminish sialorrhea but at the same time increase the chance of complications related to posterior drooling. In children with identified sensorineural hearing loss, transtympanic neurectomy would be contraindicated (Myer 1989).

REFERENCES

Arnold, H.G., Gross, C.W. (1977) 'Transtympanic neurectomy: a solution to drooling problems.' *Developmental Medicine and Child Neurology*, **19**, 509–513.

Arnrup, K., Crossner, C-G. (1990) 'Caries prevalence after submandibular duct retroposition in drooling children with neurological disorders.' *Pediatric Dentistry*, **12**, 98–101.

Bailey, C.M., Wadsworth, P.V. (1985) 'Treatment of the drooling child by submandibular duct transposition.' *Journal of Laryngology and Otology*, **99**, 1111–1117.

Blasco, P.A. (1992) 'Surgical management of drooling.' *Developmental Medicine and Child Neurology*, **34**, 368–369. *(Letter.)*

—— Stansbury, J.C.K. (1996) 'Glycopyrrolate treatment of chronic drooling.' *Archives of Pediatrics and Adolescent Medicine. (In press.)*

—— Allaire, J.H., Hollahan, J., Blasco, P.M., Edgerton, M.T., Bosma, J.F., Nowak, A.J., Sternfeld, L., McPherson, K.A., Kenny, D.J., and the participants of the Consortium on Drooling (1991) *Consensus Statement of the Consortium on Drooling.* Washington, DC: UCPA.

—— —— and participants of the Consortium on Drooling (1992) 'Drooling in the developmentally disabled: management practices and recommendations.' *Developmental Medicine and Child Neurology*, **34**, 849–862.

Bosma, J.F., Hepburn, L.G., Josell, S.D., Baker, K. (1990) 'Ultrasound demonstration of tongue motions during suckle feeding.' *Developmental Medicine and Child Neurology*, **32**, 223–229.

Boullard, K.D. (1984) 'The effectiveness of oral sensorimotor techniques in drooling reduction.' Thesis, Sargent College of Allied Health Professions, Boston University.

Brody, G.S. (1977) 'Control of drooling by translocation of parotid duct and extirpation of mandibular gland.' *Developmental Medicine and Child Neurology*, **19**, 514–517.

Brown, A.S., Silverman, J., Greenberg, S., Malamud, D.F., Album, M., Lloyd, R.W., Sarshik, M. (1985) 'A team approach to drool control in cerebral palsy.' *Annals of Plastic Surgery*, **15**, 423–430.

Brundage, S.R., Moore, W.D. (1989) 'Submandibular gland resection and bilateral parotid duct ligation as a management for chronic drooling in cerebral palsy.' *Plastic and Reconstructive Surgery*, **83**, 443–446.

Burgmayer, S., Jung, H. (1983) 'Hypersalivation in severe mental retardation.' *International Journal of Rehabilitation Research*, **6**, 193–197.

Burton, M.J. (1991) 'The surgical management of drooling.' *Developmental Medicine and Child Neurology*, **33**, 1110–1116.

Camp-Bruno, J.A., Winsberg, B.G., Green-Parsons, A.R., Abrams, J.P. (1989) 'Efficacy of benztropine therapy for drooling.' *Developmental Medicine and Child Neurology*, **31**, 309–319.

Casas, M.J., McPherson, K.A., Kenny, D.J. (1990) 'Ultrasound and electromyographic synchronization for analysis of the oral phase of swallowing in children.' *Developmental Medicine and Child Neurology*, **32**, Suppl. 62, 15. *(Abstract.)*

—— Kenny, D.J., McPherson, K.A. (1994) 'Swallowing/ventilation interactions during oral swallow in normal children and children with cerebral palsy.' *Dysphagia*, **9**, 40–46.

Creech, R.D. (1991) 'Saliva.' *In:* Blasco, P.A., Allaire, J.H., Hollahan, J., Blasco, P.M., Edgerton, M.T., Bosma, J.F., Nowak, A.J., Sternfeld, L., McPherson, K.A., Kenny, D.J., and the participants of the Consortium on Drooling *Consensus Statement of the Consortium on Drooling.* Washington, DC: UCPA, pp. 23–24.

Crysdale, W.S. (1989) 'Management options for the drooling patient.' *Ear, Nose and Throat Journal*, **68**, 820–830.

—— White A. (1989) 'Submandibular duct relocation for drooling: a 10-year experience with 194 patients.' *Otolaryngology—Head and Neck Surgery*, **101**, 87–92.

Davis, M.M., Hanke, C.W., Zollinger, T.W., Montebello, J.F., Hornback, N.B., Norins, A.L. (1989) 'Skin cancer in patients with chronic radiation dermatitis.' *Journal of the American Academy of Dermatology*, **20**, 608–616.

Dawes, C. (1978) 'The chemistry and physiology of saliva.' *In:* Shaw, J.H., Sweeney, E.A., Cappuccino, C.C.,

Meller S.M. (Eds.) *Textbook of Oral Biology.* Philadelphia: W.B. Saunders, pp. 593–616.

Drabman, R.S., Cordua Y., Cruz, G., Rosse, J., Lynd, R.S. (1979) 'Suppression of chronic drooling in mentally retarded children and adolescents: effectiveness of a behavioral treatment package.' *Behavior Therapy*, **10**, 46–56.

Dundas, D.F., Peterson, R.A. (1979) 'Surgical treatment of drooling by bilateral parotid duct ligation and submandibular gland resection.' *Plastic and Reconstructive Surgery*, **64**, 47–51.

Dunn, K.W., Cunningham, C.E., Backman, J.E. (1987) 'Self-control and reinforcement in the management of a cerebral-palsied adolescent's drooling.' *Developmental Medicine and Child Neurology*, **29**, 305–310.

Dworkin, J.P., Nadal, J.C. (1991) 'Nonsurgical treatment of drooling in a patient with closed head injury and severe dysarthria.' *Dysphagia*, **6**, 40–49.

Ekedahl, C., Månsson, I., Sandberg, N. (1974) 'Swallowing dysfunction in the brain-damaged with drooling.' *Acta Otolaryngologica*, **78**, 141–149.

Faggella, R.M., Osborn, J.M. (1983) 'Surgical correction of drool: a comparison of three groups of patients.' *Plastic and Reconstructive Surgery*, **72**, 478–482.

Fear, D.W., Hitchcock, R.P., Fonseca, R.J. (1988) 'Treatment of chronic drooling: a preliminary report.' *Oral Surgery, Oral Medicine, and Oral Pathology*, **66**, 163–166.

Garber, N.B. (1971) 'Operant procedures to eliminate drooling behavior in a cerebral palsied adolescent.' *Developmental Medicine and Child Neurology*, **13**, 641–644.

Goode, R.L., Smith, R.A. (1970) 'The surgical management of sialorrhea.' *Laryngoscope*, **80**, 1078–1089.

Gross, C.W. (1990) 'Surgical management of sialorrhea.' *Otolaryngology—Head and Neck Surgery*, **103**, 671. (*Letter.*)

Guerin, R.L. (1979) 'Surgical management of drooling.' *Archives of Otolaryngology*, **105**, 535–537.

Haberfellner, H., Rossiwall, B. (1977) 'Treatment of oral sensorimotor disorders in cerebral-palsied children: preliminary report.' *Developmental Medicine and Child Neurology*, **19**, 350–352.

Harris, M.M., Dignam, P.F. (1980) 'A non-surgical method of reducing drooling in cerebral-palsied children.' *Developmental Medicine and Child Neurology*, **22**, 293–299.

Hotaling, A.J., Madgy, D.N., Kuhns, L.R., Filipek, L., Belenky, W.M. (1992) 'Postoperative technetium scanning in patients with submandibular duct diversion.' *Archives of Otolaryngology, Head and Neck Surgery*, **118**, 1331–1333.

Johnson, H., Scott, A. (Eds.) (1993) *A Practical Approach to Saliva Control.* Tucson, AZ: Communication/ Therapy Skill Builders.

Jones, B. (1993) 'Behavior management.' *In:* Johnson, H., Scott, A. (Eds.) *A Practical Approach to Saliva Control.* Tucson, AZ: Communication/Therapy Skill Builders, pp. 44–55.

Jones, P.R. (1982) 'The Meldreth dribble control project reassessed.' *Child: Care, Health, and Development*, **8**, 65–75.

Kaplan, M.D., Baum, B.J. (1993) 'The functions of saliva.' *Dysphagia*, **8**, 225–229.

Koheil, R., Sochaniwskyj, A.E., Bablich, K., Kenny, D.J., Milner, M. (1987) 'Biofeedback techniques and behaviour modification in the conservative remediation of drooling by children with cerebral palsy.' *Developmental Medicine and Child Neurology*, **29**, 19–26.

Lashley, K.S. (1917) 'Changes in the amount of salivary secretion associated with cerebral lesions.' *American Journal of Physiology*, **43**, 62–72.

Lespargot, A., Langevin, M-F., Muller, S., Guillemont, S. (1993) 'Swallowing disturbances associated with drooling in cerebral-palsied children.' *Developmental Medicine and Child Neurology*, **35**, 298–304.

Lewis, D.W., Fontana, C., Mehallick, L.K., Everett, Y. (1994) 'Transdermal scopolamine for reduction of drooling in developmentally delayed children.' *Developmental Medicine and Child Neurology*, **36**, 484–486.

Limbrock, G.J., Hoyer, H., Scheying, H. (1990) 'Drooling, chewing and swallowing dysfunctions in children with cerebral palsy: treatment according to Castillo-Morales.' *Journal of Dentistry for Children*, **57**, 445–451.

Lipkin, P. (1991) 'Epidemiology of the developmental disabilities.' *In:* Capute, A.J., Accardo, P.J. (Eds.) *Developmental Disabilities in Infancy and Childhood.* Baltimore: Paul Brookes, pp. 43–67.

Lourie, R.S. (1943) 'Rate of secretion of the parotid glands in normal children. A measurement of function of the autonomic nervous system.' *American Journal of Diseases of Children*, **65**, 455–479.

Martin, H., Strong, E., Spiro, R.H. (1970) 'Radiation-induced skin cancer of the head and neck.' *Cancer*, **25**, 61–71.

Michel, R.G., Johnson, K.A., Patterson, C.N. (1977) 'Parasympathetic nerve section for control of sialorrhea.' *Archives of Otolaryngology*, **103**, 94–97.

103

Mullins, W.M., Gross, C.W., Moore, J.M. (1979) 'Long-term follow-up of tympanic neurectomy for sialorrhea.' *Laryngoscope*, **89**, 1219–1223.

Myer, C.M. (1989) 'Sialorrhea.' *Pediatric Clinics of North America*, **36**, 1495–1500.

Nelson, E.C., Pendleton, T.B., Edel, J. (1981) 'Lip halter. An aid in drool control.' *Physical Therapy*, **61**, 361–362.

Ottenbacher, K., Bundy, A., Short, M.A. (1983) 'The development and treatment of oral-motor dysfunction: a review of clinical research.' *Physical and Occupational Therapy in Pediatrics*, **3**, 147–160.

Pogrel, M.A. (1987) 'Sialodochoplasty—does it work?' *International Journal of Oral and Maxillofacial Surgery*, **16**, 266–269.

Prentice, J. (1991) 'Salivary overflow.' *In:* Blasco, P.A., Allaire, J.H., Hollahan, J., Blasco, P.M., Edgerton, M.T., Bosma, J.F., Nowak, A.J., Sternfeld, L., McPherson, K.A., Kenny, D.J., and the participants of the Consortium on Drooling (1991) *Consensus Statement of the Consortium on Drooling.* Washington, DC: UCPA, pp. 22–23.

Rapp, D. (1980) 'Drool control: long-term follow-up.' *Developmental Medicine and Child Neurology*, **22**, 448–453.

Reddihough, D., Johnson, H., Staples, M., Hudson, I., Exarchos, H. (1990) 'Use of benzhexol hydrochloride to control drooling of children with cerebral palsy.' *Developmental Medicine and Child Neurology*, **32**, 985–989.

Richman, J.S., Kozlowski, N.L. (1977) 'Operant training of head control and beginning language for a severely developmentally disabled child.' *Journal of Behavior Therapy and Experimental Psychiatry*, **8**, 437–440.

Rosen, A., Komisar, A., Ophir, D., Marshak, G. (1990) 'Experience with the Wilkie procedure for sialorrhea.' *Annals of Otology, Rhinology, and Laryngology*, **99**, 730–732.

Schneyer, L.H., Levin, L.K. (1954) 'Rate of flow of "resting" saliva from individual gland pairs in man.' *Journal of Dental Research*, **33**, 716–717. *(Abstract.)*

Sellars, S.L. (1985) 'Surgery of sialorrhoea.' *Journal of Laryngology and Otology*, **99**, 1107–1109.

Shavell, A. (1977) 'Drooling in cerebral palsy.' *South African Journal of Communication Disorders*, **24**, 75–88.

Shott, S.R., Myer, C.M., Cotton, R.T. (1989) 'Surgical management of sialorrhea.' *Otolaryngology—Head and Neck Surgery*, **101**, 47–50.

Siegel, L.K., Klingbeil, M.A. (1991) 'Control of drooling with transdermal scopolamine in a child with cerebral palsy.' *Developmental Medicine and Child Neurology*, **33**, 1013–1014.

Smith, W.L., Erenberg, A., Nowak, A., Franken, E.A. (1985) 'Physiology of sucking in the normal term infant using real-time US.' *Radiology*, **156**, 379–381.

Sochaniwskyj, A.E. (1982) 'Drool quantification: noninvasive technique.' *Archives of Physical Medicine and Rehabilitation*, **63**, 605–607.

—— Koheil, R.M., Bablich, K., Milner, M., Kenny, D.J. (1986) 'Oral motor functioning, frequency of swallowing and drooling in normal children and in children with cerebral palsy.' *Archives of Physical Medicine and Rehabilitation*, **67**, 866–874.

Stevenson, R.D., Allaire, J.H., Blasco, P.A. (1994) 'Deterioration of feeding behavior following surgical treatment of drooling.' *Dysphagia*, **9**, 22–25.

Talmi, Y.P., Finkelstein, Y., Zohar, Y. (1990) 'Reduction of salivary flow with transdermal scopolamine: a four-year experience.' *Otolaryngology—Head and Neck Surgery*, **103**, 615–618.

Thorbecke, P.J., Jackson, H.J. (1982) 'Reducing chronic drooling in a retarded female using a multi-treatment package.' *Journal of Behavior Therapy and Experimental Psychiatry*, **13**, 89–93.

Toremalm, N.G., Bjerre, I. (1976) 'Surgical elimination of drooling.' *Laryngoscope*, **86**, 104–112.

Trott, M.C., Maechtlen, A.D. (1986) 'The use of overcorrection as a means to control drooling.' *American Journal of Occupational Therapy*, **40**, 702–704.

US Department of Health and Human Services (1989) *Oral Complications of Cancer Therapies: Diagnosis, Prevention, and Treatment.* Bethesda, MD: NIH Consensus Development Conference, Office of Medical Applications of Research.

Vaughan, J.M. (1971) 'The effects of radiation on bone.' *In:* Bourne, G.H. (Ed.) *The Biochemistry and Physiology of Bone, 2nd Edn.* New York: Academic Press, pp. 485–534.

Vice, F.L., Heinz, J.M., Giuriati, G., Hood, M., Bosma, J.F. (1990) 'Cervical auscultation of suckle feeding in newborn infants.' *Developmental Medicine and Child Neurology*, **32**, 760–768.

Weiner, N. (1980) 'Atropine, scopolamine, and related antimuscarinic drugs.' *In:* Gilman, A.G., Goodman, L.S., Gilman, A. (Eds.) *The Pharmacological Basis of Therapeutics, 6th Edn.* New York: MacMillan, pp. 120–137.

Weiss-Lambrou, R., Tétreault, S., Dudley, J. (1988) 'The relationship between oral sensation and drooling in persons with cerebral palsy.' *American Journal of Occupational Therapy*, **43**, 155–161.

Wilkie, T.F., Brody, G.S. (1977) 'The surgical treatment of drooling. A ten-year review.' *Plastic and Reconstructive Surgery*, **59**, 791–798.

Wilkinson, J.A. (1987) 'Side effects of transdermal scopolamine.' *Journal of Emergency Medicine*, **5**, 389–392.

Williams, M.B. (1991) 'Meditations on the Wet Stuff.' *In:* Blasco, P.A., Allaire, J.H., Hollahan, J., Blasco, P.M., Edgerton, M.T., Bosma, J.F., Nowak, A.J., Sternfeld, L., McPherson, K.A., Kenny, D.J., and the participants of the Consortium on Drooling (1991) *Consensus Statement of the Consortium on Drooling.* Washington, DC: UCPA, pp. 21–22.

Ziskind, A.A. (1988) 'Transdermal scopolamine-induced psychosis.' *Postgraduate Medicine*, **84**, 73–76.

ACKNOWLEDGEMENTS

The participants of the Consortium on Drooling held in Charlottesville, VA, July 10–11, 1990, were essential to the development of this information. I gratefully acknowledge also the assistance and contributions of the following people: Bruce Baker, Joan Bergman, James A. Blackman, Patricia M. Blasco, James F. Bosma, Richard Dodds, Milton T. Edgerton, Frank Farmer, Catherine L. Fox, Risa Gressard, Charles W. Gross, Joyce M. Hillstrom, James Hollahan, Sharon L. Hostler, David J. Kenny, Carol Long, Karen McPherson, F. Don Nidiffer, Arthur J. Nowak, Barbara M. Rhodes, Barry A. Romich, Niti Singh, Leon Sternfeld, Judy Widder and Daniel L. Winfield.

10
CONSTIPATION IN DISABLED CHILDREN

Graham Clayden

Difficulty with defaecation is a common problem for children who have other disabilities. Recognition and therefore effective management is often delayed because the other disabilities eclipse those related to defaecation. This may be due to the importance to health or survival of these other problems, such as poor nutrition, airway difficulties, recurrent infections, seizures or sensory deficiencies. However, disregard of the defaecation problems may result from parental embarrassment, professional delicacy or low expectation. Even though these bowel problems are rarely life-threatening they do contribute to reduction of the quality of life for the disabled person (Thomas *et al.* 1989) and reduce the chance of families managing the child at home.

Definition

The term *constipation* has no clear definition and appears to be used by some to describe the hardness of stools and by others to indicate an unreasonable delay in defaecation. In this chapter the term is used to describe a delay in defaecation beyond the normal range which leads to distress to the child or carer (Clayden 1976). This distress may be abdominal pain and anal discomfort when an accumulated and hard stool is imminent or being passed. It may arise from the carers having to cope with overflow faecal incontinence or the child suffering from the resulting perianal soreness. Many parents and other carers report an aggravation of a number of other problems with increasingly long intervals between stools. Some children lose their already poor appetites when constipated (Clayden 1994*a*), others have more convulsions, or show a deterioration of behaviour or concentration. The loaded rectum may distort the bladder, leading to compromised urinary continence and frequent urinary tract infections (Friedmann 1968, O'Regan *et al.* 1985, Yazbeck *et al.* 1987).

Most children open their bowels between three times per day and once in every three days (Connell *et al.* 1965, Weaver 1988). Intervals of longer than three days should not necessarily lead to investigation or active treatment but should alert everyone to explore carefully whether this delay is exaggerating some of the other features of the disability or creating a vicious cycle.

High risk of constipation

Constipation may arise because of abnormalities in: consistency of the stool; motility of the lower bowel; size and position of the anus; reflex relaxation of the internal anal sphincter; competence of the voluntary muscles involved; sensation from the anorectum; perception of this sensation; or behavioural response to the need to defaecate. Many disabilities in children are associated with an increased likelihood of these abnormalities either solely or in combination. It may be helpful to expand this list by considering each factor with some of the more common disabling conditions.

Consistency of the stool
The consistency of a stool depends on its fibre and fluid content. The child's diet will therefore dictate the type of stool formed. A large number of children with cerebral palsy have difficulties in eating and drinking in early life. When on the brink of failing to thrive, every consideration must be given to achieving maximum calorie intake. Fibre must take second place to more nutritious foods when intake is limited by chewing and swallowing difficulties as is seen in cerebral palsy. However, a balance must be achieved to prevent the development of a vicious cycle where the constipation causes abdominal pain related to eating as a result of the gastrocolic reflex provoking a colonic contraction onto hard retained faeces and so adding to the feeding difficulty.

Motility of the lower bowel
Intestinal motility may be abnormal in children with disorders affecting the myenteric plexus or the smooth muscle of the bowel. Conditions such as neurofibromatosis (Feinstat *et al.* 1984) or multiple endocrine neoplasia type 2b are associated with ganglioneuromatosis of the bowel and may present with severe colonic dysmotility (Carney *et al.* 1976). Myotonic dystrophy (Harper 1975, Eckardt and Nix 1991) and later stages of muscular dystrophy are associated with deteriorating colorectal motility. The abnormality of the anal sphincter may lead to confusion with the signs of sexual abuse especially in myotonic dystrophy (Reardon *et al.* 1992) which is particularly difficult to assess given the increased risk of sexual abuse in disabled children (Thomas *et al.* 1989). Endocrine and metabolic abnormalities such as hypothyroidism and hypercalcaemia are associated with constipation mainly through slow transit, although the water demands in hypercalcaemia add to the drying of the stool.

Exercise appears to stimulate intestinal motility and this then is another way in which children with immobility have an increased risk of constipation. A large number of children who have complex special needs are on medication. Many drugs have an effect on intestinal motility. It is very common for children with a tendency to constipation to have a major relapse when given a simple cough linctus. Many anticonvulsants and phenothiazines are constipating (Loening-Baucke 1993).

Size and position of the anus
A number of syndromes are associated with abnormal development of the anorectum. The embryology of the hind gut is complex and so anomalies are relatively common and are frequently associated with those of the urinary tract. The anus is derived from an ectodermal indenting to meet the rectal part of the cloaca. The dividing anorectal membrane normally disappears by the eighth postconceptional week, although remnants can be detected by neonatal rectal examination in a large number of children (5 per cent of boys and 23 per cent of girls) (Harris *et al.* 1954). Imperforate anus and anal stenosis are associated with constipation and a degree of incontinence even with early and effective surgical correction. Minor degrees of anal stenosis or stricture may go unnoticed (Kiely *et al.* 1979) and should

always be considered if straining to pass stools starts in infancy and an eventual passage of a thin ribbon-shaped stool is described.

Reflex relaxation of the internal anal sphincter
The internal anal sphincter has a normal resting squeeze pressure of about 30 mmHg. When a stool moves into the rectum as a result of the motility of the colon, the rectum contracts down onto the stool producing a wave of pressure lasting about 5 seconds. The anal pressure drops simultaneously, thus allowing the stool to descend. This recto-anal reflex is transmitted via the myenteric plexus which is effectively absent in Hirschsprung's disease due to a failure of migration and penetration by the neuroblasts arising from the cervical neural crest in the embryo. It is not surprising that Hirschsprung's disease presents with neonatal intestinal obstruction if a long segment is aganglionic. However, if the segment deficient of myenteric plexus ganglion cells is short, constipation may present later. Although Hirschsprung's disease is not commonly associated with other syndromes it is 10 times more common in Down syndrome than in children with a normal karyotype (Passarge 1967).

Even in the child with normal ganglion cells, recto-anal reflex relaxation of the anal sphincter may not be completed until high rectal volumes of faeces are present when the child has or develops a megarectum. In this situation the child has a bag-shaped rectum (instead of the usual folded tube) which fills with progressively hardening stools but allowing lose stool to slip past the faecal ball and escape through the partially inhibited anal sphincter to produce virtually continuous liquid soiling. Occasionally the child passes a massive (and usually very painful) stool which leads to a few days remission from the soiling. However, the pain experienced teaches the child that defaecation should be avoided at all costs and the capacity of the megarectum permits the child to do this. This produces a vicious cycle of constipation. The prevention of a megarectum is an important step in the management of constipation and is a major indication for early and effective treatment.

Competence of the voluntary muscles involved
Defaecation depends on coordinated voluntary (striated) muscle function and coordination as well as the rectoanal inhibitory reflex. The coordination of external sphincter relaxation, levator ani stabilization of the anus, abdominal muscle contraction and grunting is a reflex activity in infants but gradually comes under voluntary control in the second year of life. This allows the achievement of socially acceptable continence by the age of 3 years in the majority of children (Butler and Golding 1986). For children—such as those with spina bifida—who have deficiency of the spinal nerves and so lack control of these muscles, faecal continence is difficult to achieve (Lie et al. 1991, Agnarsson et al. 1993a). Not only do they have a problem delaying defaecation owing to poor sensation and the weakness of the external sphincter, but they also have an exaggerated inhibitory reflex of the internal anal sphincter (Arhan et al. 1984). This means that any stool in the rectum will completely inhibit the anal tone. The absence of effective external sphincter severely limits the chance of continence (Chantraine et al. 1966).

The problem can also be compounded by constipation. Martin Bax (personal communication) reports that 67 per cent of young people with spina bifida had problems with constipation

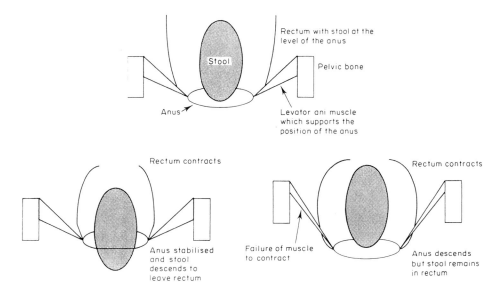

Fig. 10.1. Diagram showing the relative movement of stool in healthy children *(lower left)* and in children with spina bifida *(lower right)*. (Reproduced by permission from Buchanan 1993.)

and 42 per cent were still having manual evacuations performed even into adolescence either by themselves or by a parent. Constipation may occur in children with a neuropathic bowel as a result of poor sensation of rectal filling and rectal fullness and by the instability of the position of the anus during rectal contraction (Clayden 1992*a*).

Figure 10.1 illustrates the problem. During rectal contraction the anus should be stabilized by the levator ani muscles. Failure to achieve this allows the anus to move distally with the stool which therefore fails to leave the rectum before the rectal contraction ceases. It is the equivalent to a person trying to leave a room through a door which opens outwards but is set in an elastic wall. Pressure to open the door is met with the doorway moving further away making evacuation difficult. Persistent failure to complete defaecation in infancy may encourage the rectum to grow larger, as is the case with any partially obstructed viscus. This increases the mechanical difficulties as the stools are then larger and more difficult to evacuate through the unstable anus, and overflow faecal soiling adds to the childs' incontinence.

If a megarectum can be prevented by early care to ensure regular defaecation and avoidance of constipation by regular lavatory visits and the use of methods to complete defaecation, future faecal continence is likely to be achieved. In the absence of megarectum, antimotility drugs such as codeine phosphate or loperamide can be used to suppress the moment of defaecation until socially more easily coped with. Once a degree of megarectum has developed, continence will only be achieved if the large rectum can be emptied completely at a socially convenient time. This usually involves the use of enemas which are

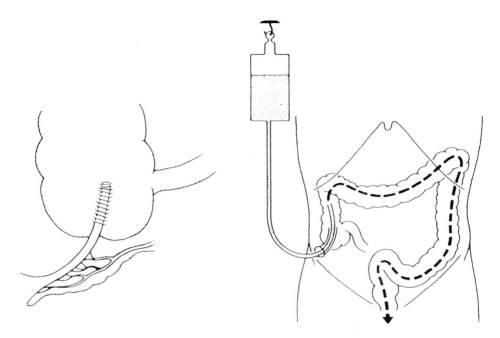

Fig. 10.2. Diagram showing the anatomical position of the antegrade continence enema (ACE) in the Malone procedure. (Reproduced by permission from Malone *et al.* 1990.)

fortunately painless as a result of the sensory loss. However, they are difficult to administer effectively. The rapid inhibition of the anal sphincter caused by the rectal distension with the enema fluid makes an effective evacuation of a loaded bowel difficult depending on the degree of the loading. Special continence catheters which plug the anus are available (Shandling and Gilmour 1987), as are stoma washout kits where conical plugs are incorporated into the tip of the catheter. There are problems for children to perform these evacuation techniques independently especially if they have to try to balance on the lavatory at the same time.

A small operation has been devised to allow effective flushing of the bowel without having to resort to trying to plug the anus at the same time as filling the rectum with fluid. By applying the Metrofanoff procedure to the bowel problem, Malone *et al.* (1990) pioneered the formation of a continent stoma by using the appendix, as shown in Figure 10.2. This allows a catheter to be passed into the ascending colon through the appendicostomy where fluids can be flushed in to evacuate the distal bowel. This allows the child to be continent as there is no residual stool in the rectum. Most children require the antegrade colonic enema (ACE) every 48 hours to maintain continence. The choice of flushing fluid depends on the original degree of megarectum: phosphate enema is often used but may produce problems with a major degree of faecal retention; polyethylene glycol solution ('Klean-Prep') on its own or with bisacodyl enema solution is effective.

110

Sensation from the anorectum

More minor neurological loss may effect the sensation of rectal fullness and the urgency of defaecation only. A number of children have reasonable anal sphincter activity when tested but have a poor appreciation of the need to defaecate. They can be helped by developing a regular pattern of timed use of the lavatory and by avoiding faecal retention. Poor sensation may also be a consequence of a megarectum. The sensation arises in the rectum when the stretch receptors are activated. An average size stool joining the rectal faecal mass in a megarectum is hardly noticed and merely adds to the obstructing megastool and to the overflow faecal soiling.

Perception of rectal sensation

As part of their achieving faecal continence, children learn to recognize the sensation of rectal fullness and therefore their chances of success if they visit the lavatory or pot. With practice they become more sophisticated in their ability to differentiate flatus from fluid from faeces as well as judging the urgency of the situation. Their success in the acquisition of these important social skills will depend on the degree of rectal sensation, the consistency of the faeces (delayed with loose stools), the consistency of their training to use the lavatory/pot, and their learning ability/developmental stage. No-one expects a 6-month-old baby to be continent, but one would hope that a child by 3 years is having few incontinent accidents. It may be difficult to judge when a child with learning difficulties should be able to use the lavatory effectively—perhaps the easiest guide is when she reaches the developmental age of 3 years. There is good evidence that, provided sufficient resources are provided for effective behavioural psychological help, many more children with severe learning difficulties could be continent (Smith *et al.* 1994). Once again the presence of constipation will sabotage training for faecal continence.

Behavioural response to the need to defaecate

Once the child has perceived the need to defaecate, the decision to do so will depend on the child's experience. If previous episodes of defaecation have resulted in severe anal pain or parental disgust, the child is likely to attempt to avoid it. Constipation becomes a vicious cycle mainly as a result of these two experiences. For children with special needs, pain or shame may be even more difficult to tolerate than for ordinary children in proportion to their degree of communication difficulty. Pain during defaecation for a child with cerebral palsy is likely to provoke a muscle spasm which may involve the external sphincter and other pelvic floor muscles. This may lead to a contraction of the anal muscles onto a partially expelled stool leading to even more pain and resulting fear.

Children who fail to achieve reasonable toileting skills feel themselves failures and have a low self-esteem. This may be aggravated by the use of painful and humiliating treatments such as enemas and suppositories. Many normally mobile children, when faced with an experience of which they are afraid, will run off or hide. It is a frequent report that constipated children who feel that the dreaded stool is imminent will hide and seek solitude. Children who are immobile are unable to express their fears in this way and so are probably more vulnerable to the feelings of fear and helplessness. Their fear of defaecation is exceeded only by their fear of anal procedures (unless there is sensory loss as in most children with spina bifida). Ignoring the child's fear is not only heartless and unprofessional but may consolidate the resistance to defaecation and increase the risk of dissociation for any rectal sensation.

Managing the bowel problem in a disabled child
As can be seen from the factors leading to ineffective defaecation, there are a number of principles involved in helping disabled children that are true for all children but are emphasized because of the disabled child's increased vulnerability.

Assessment
It should be possible to ascertain from the history whether the main problem is a failure to achieve faecal continence or whether constipation is leading to an overflow incontinence. Normal consistency stools are passed in the nappy or randomly in clothes once or twice per day in the former case. However, with constipation and overflow incontinence, frequent loose or semi-solid faeces are passed often with a history of episodes of remission following the passage of a very large stool. The age of onset of constipation is one of the best guides to whether there is an anorectal anomaly or Hirschsprung's disease, when onset is as a young infant in contrast to problems presenting around pot training.

Faeces are usually palpable on abdominal examination if there is any degree of megarectum, unless the stools remain very soft as is the case when the child is on a particularly high fibre diet.

Investigations may be necessary to be certain of the diagnosis of the bowel disorder. Any suggestion of Hirschsprung's disease should lead to a suction rectal biopsy and histochemical examination for excessive acetylcholinesterase positive nerves. Any doubt about the degree of faecal retention can be resolved by performing an abdominal radiograph four or five days after the child swallows a series of radio-opaque markers taken on days 1, 2 and 3. The markers can be seen on the abdominal radiograph and can give valuable evidence of slow colonic transit as well as the degree of retention in the rectum and some idea of its size (Arhan *et al.* 1981). Anorectal manometry has been shown to give valuable evidence of the neuropathic rectum and an estimate of the sensory deficit in children with spina bifida and other spinal cord problems (Agnarsson *et al.* 1993*a*). It can also be used as a form of biofeedback where rectal sensation and the perception of the feelings is inefficient (Whitehead *et al.* 1986, Loening-Baucke *et al.* 1988). Anorectal manometry is probably of little value in children with cerebral palsy (Agnarsson *et al.* 1993*b*, Staiano and Del Giudice 1994).

Treatment
The basic principles for the treatment of constipation need to be applied for disabled children as for other children (Clayden 1992*b*, Loening-Baucke 1993). They can be summarized as follows.
• *Prevention.* Establish an experience of easy pain-free defaecation from as early in life as possible by providing a diet with plenty of fluid and fibre. This is a particular problem

with children with feeding difficulties but a compromise between nutrition and fibre can be reached by using high nutrition/high fibre special foods. Another important area of prevention of constipation is the early recognition of anal discomfort in children and the avoidance of aggravating the pain by careless rectal procedures or treatments when other routes are possible. A number of children have local perianal skin infection with group A *Streptococcus* rather than the commoner anal fissure. Antibiotics in addition to regular stool softeners are essential.

• *Select the treatment for the degree of faecal retention.* A stimulant laxative given to a grossly faecally impacted child will produce abdominal colic and an increase in watery over-flow incontinence. An enema forced on a frightened deliberately faecally retaining child may prolong the period of retention for years (Pinkerton 1958). Treatment can only be selected after careful assessment and with knowledge of what will be tolerated or complied with. This is a particularly important principle for children with learning difficulties.

• *Inform.* Careful education is essential to explain to the child, parents and colleagues the pathophysiology and the reasons behind the various management schemes. A clear statement of the problems and the details of treatment should be shared. This will prevent confusion by reducing conflicting advice.

• *Softening.* All retained stools need to be softened. Sometimes that is all that is required: the softened stool is spontaneously passed and the obstruction episode is over. Stools can be softened using docusate sodium (Dioctyl paediatric syrup to a maximum of 2 ml/kg/day). Sometimes lactulose may be sufficient or even addition of extra fruit juice.

• *Evacuation.* Fortunately a number of children will clear their residual rectal faecal collection after a week or two on docusate. For those who do not, an escalating regime may be used tailored to the child's needs and sensitivities. If a small soft faecal collection is palpable abdominally, a reasonable dose of senna may clear it. If the stool is soft but larger it may be necessary to give sodium picosulphate either as the elixir or in sachet form. If this fails to clear the stool then the following day the child could be given either a phosphate enema or sodium citrate micro-enema by a skilled and trusted nurse or else polyethylene glycol solution ('Klean-Prep') provided the child is able to drink the required 1 to 2 litres of re-constituted solution. Some children vomit this volume and may need an antiemetic simul-taneously (Koletzko *et al.* 1989). Some authorities recommend giving polyethylene glycol via a nasogastric tube but this may be more distressing than an enema and much less ex-plicable to the child with learning difficulties.

If these medical methods fail then an evacuation of faeces under a general anaesthetic may be necessary. If there is gross impaction, especially with urinary retention, a manual evacuation is necessary. Unfortunately the disabled child may have a higher risk from the anaesthesia and this must be taken into consideration when deciding on the means of evacu-ation. There is some evidence that in the presence of a megarectum the anal sphincter is less responsive to the inhibitory reflex. This is the rationale behind a vigorous anal dilatation that can be performed under the same anaesthetic as the evacuation.

• *Maintenance laxatives.* Stimulant laxatives are usually necessary in any child with a degree of megarectum. Standardized senna ('Senokot') is an easily titratable preparation depending on severity of the constipation tendency. It is best given in a single daily dose but increasing the dose incrementally until effective. When there is a poor fibre intake a stool bulking agent such as methylcellulose, lactulose or bran is helpful. Many children who appear to be opening their bowels more regularly on senna gradually accumulate stool in their large rectums. A weekend dose of sodium picosulphate or even polyethylene glycol solution may prevent a major relapse. One of the greatest problems is the reluctance of parents to continue the maintenance laxatives for long enough. Theirs is an understandable anxiety in response to advice to avoid unnecessary laxatives in children. This is very good evidence of the need to provide parents with full information and to help them to understand the indications for the treatments (Clayden and Agnarsson 1991).

The medical and surgical treatments will fail, even if given diligently and with the maximum of careful education, unless *psychological factors* in the cause and persistence of the bowel problem are addressed. The role of fear and helplessness has been discussed, but sometimes these feelings become enmeshed with the other emotions within the child and the family (Clayden 1994*b*). In the child with complex medical needs, the bowel problem may be the tangible centre for the family's rejection of this problem child. Discussions about the distress of incontinence may gravitate to remind the parents and the child of their underlying and sometimes denied deeper distress at the overall disability. All parents lose their temper about faecal incontinence at some stage and feel very guilty later. This guilt may awaken the guilt about producing an 'incomplete' child and suddenly become unbearable. For all these reasons, those helping children and families with these distressing and socially isolating bowel problems need a fully supportive network. This network should include child psychologists, psychiatrists, nurse specialists and psychiatric social workers who should share with the other clinicians a common model of the child's particular needs.

Conclusion
Although constipation and faecal incontinence are particularly difficult to manage in children with other disabilities, it is essential that they are clearly recorded in the problem list. Early treatment may prevent the development of a megarectum or an established fear of defaecation and so they should not be relegated to a category of 'to be considered later'. The challenge to the clinician is to temper the enthusiasm or the desperation to use intensive or invasive treatment regimes with a balanced empathetic assessment of the meaning of the bowel problem to the child. A major operation for the relief of recurrent constipation with episodes of severe abdominal and anal pain may be justified for the child's sake especially when faecal loading is associated with aggravation of other medical problems. However, considerable care must be taken in making similar decisions for the management of faecal incontinence which may produce no discomfort for the child but be very distressing for the carer. Sometimes a surgical option appears to offer the most rapid solution, but in the situation where the patient is incompetent to give personal consent, the clinician must seek what will genuinely benefit the child. Obviously the parental distress must be seriously considered out of fairness to them as well as to preserve the stability of the place in the family home for the disabled child. However, a great deal can be done to relieve this burden for them by providing expert continence advisors and financial support for continence aids in addition to access to clinicians who take these problems seriously.

REFERENCES

Agnarsson, U., Warde, C., McCarthy, G., Clayden, G.S., Evans, N. (1993a) 'Anorectal function of children with neurological problems. I: Spina bifida.' *Developmental Medicine and Child Neurology*, **35**, 893–902.

—— —— —— —— —— (1993b) 'Anorectal function of children with neurological problems. II: Cerebral palsy.' *Developmental Medicine and Child Neurology*, **35**, 903–980.

Arhan, P., Devroede, G., Jehannin, B., Lanza, M., Faverdin, C., Dornic, C., Persoz, B., Tétreault, L., Perey, B., Pellerin, D. (1981) 'Segmental colonic transit time.' *Diseases of the Colon and Rectum*, **24**, 625–629.

—— Faverdin, C., Devroede, G., Pierre-Kahn, A., Scott, H., Pellerin, D. (1984) 'Anorectal motility after surgery for spina bifida.' *Diseases of the Colon and Rectum*, **27**, 159–163.

Butler, N.R., Golding, J. (1986) *From Birth to Five: a Study of the Health and Behaviour of Britain's 5-year-olds.* Oxford: Pergamon.

Carney, J.A., Go, V.L.W., Sizemore, G.W., Hayles, A.B. (1976) 'Alimentary-tract ganglioneuromatosis. A major component of the syndrome of multiple endocrine neoplasia, type 2b.' *New England Journal of Medicine*, **295**, 1287–1291.

Chantraine, A., Lloyd, K., Swinyard, C.A. (1966) 'The sphincter ani externus in spina bifida and myelomeningocele.' *Journal of Urology*, **95**, 250–256.

Clayden, G.S. (1976) 'Constipation and soiling in childhood.' *British Medical Journal*, **1**, 515–517.

—— (1992a) 'Neurological disorders and faecal incontinence.' *In:* Buchanan, A. (Ed.) *Children Who Soil.* Chichester: John Wiley, pp. 158–166.

—— (1992b) 'Management of chronic constipation.' *Archives of Disease in Childhood*, **67**, 340–344.

—— (1994a) 'Clinical features of idiopathic megarectum and megacolon in children.' *In:* Kamm, M.A., Lennard-Jones, J.E. (Eds.) *Constipation.* Petersfield, Hampshire: Wrightson Biomedical, pp. 219–224.

—— (1994b) 'Constipation as a behavioural problem in children.' *In:* Kamm, M.A., Lennard-Jones, J.E. (Eds.) *Constipation.* Petersfield, Hampshire: Wrightson Medical, pp. 117–122.

—— Agnarsson, U. (1991) *Constipation in Childhood.* Oxford: Oxford University Press.

Connell, A.M., Hilton, C., Irvine, G., Lennard-Jones, J.E., Misiewicz, J.J. (1965) 'Variation of bowel habit in two population samples'. *British Medical Journal*, **2**, 1095–1099.

Eckardt, V.F., Nix, W. (1991) 'The anal sphincter in patients with myotonic muscular dystrophy.' *Gastroenterology*, **100**, 424–430.

Feinstat, T., Tesluk, H., Schuffler, M.D., Krishnamurthy, S., Verlenden, L., Gilles, W., Frey, C., Trudeau, W. (1984) 'Megacolon and neurofibromatosis: a neuronal intestinal dysplasia. Case report and review of the literature.' *Gastroenterology*, **86**, 1573–1579.

Friedmann, C.A. (1968) 'The action of nicotine and catecholamines on the human internal anal sphincter.' *American Journal of Digestive Diseases*, **13**, 428–431.

Harper, P.S. (1975) 'Congenital myotonic dystrophy in Britain. I: Clinical aspects.' *Archives of Disease in Childhood*, **50**, 505–513.

Harris, L.E., Corbin, H.P.F., Hill, J.R. (1954) 'Anorectal rings in infancy: incidence and significance.' *Pediatrics*, **13**, 59–63.

Kiely, E.M., Chopra, R., Corkery, J.J. (1979) 'Delayed diagnosis of congenital anal stenosis.' *Archives of Disease in Childhood*, **54**, 68–70.

Koletzko, S., Stringer, D.A., Cleghorn, G.J., Durie, P.R. (1989) 'Lavage treatment of distal intestinal obstruction syndrome in children with cystic fibrosis.' *Pediatrics*, **83**, 727–733.

Loening-Baucke, V. (1993) 'Chronic constipation in children.' *Gastroenterology*, **105**, 1557–1564.

—— Desch, L., Wolraich, M. (1988) 'Biofeedback training with patients with myelomeningocele and fecal incontinence.' *Developmental Medicine and Child Neurology*, **30**, 781–790.

Lie, H.R., Lagergren, J., Rasmussen, F., Lagerkvist, B., Hagelsteen, J., Börjeson, M-C., Muttilainen, M., Taudorf, K. (1991) 'Bowel and bladder control of children with myelomeningocele: a Nordic study.' *Developmental Medicine and Child Neurology*, **33**, 1053–1061.

Malone, P.S., Ransley, P.G., Kiely, E.M. (1990) 'Preliminary report: the antegrade continence enema.' *Lancet*, **336**, 1217–1218.

O'Regan, S., Yazbeck, S., Schick, E. (1985) 'Constipation, bladder instability, urinary tract infection syndrome.' *Clinical Nephrology*, **23**, 152–154.

Passarge, E. (1967) 'The genetics of Hirschsprung's disease. Evidence for heterogenous etiology and a study of sixty-three families.' *New England Journal of Medicine*, **276**, 138–143.

Pinkerton, P. (1958) 'Psychogenic megacolon in children: the implications of bowel negativism.' *Archives of Disease in Childhood*, **33**, 371–380.

Reardon, W., Hughes, H.E., Green, S.H., Lloyd Woolley, V., Harper, P.S. (1992) 'Anal abnormalities in childhood myotonic dystrophy - a possible source of confusion in child sexual abuse.' *Archives of Disease in Childhood*, **67**, 527–528.

Shandling, B., Gilmour, R.F. (1987) 'The enema continence catheter in spina bifida: successful bowel management.' *Journal of Pediatric Surgery*, **22**, 271–273.

Smith, L.J., Franchetti, B., McCoull, K., Pattison, D., Pickstock, J. (1994) 'A behavioural approach to retraining bowel function after long-standing constipation and faecal impaction in people with learning disabilities.' *Developmental Medicine and Child Neurology*, **36**, 41–49.

Staiano, A., Del Giudice, E. (1994) 'Colonic transit and anorectal manometry in children with severe brain damage.' *Pediatrics*, **94**, 169–173.

Thomas, A.P., Bax, M.C.O., Smyth, D.P.L. (1989) *The Health and Social Needs of Young Adults with Physical Disabilities. Clinics in Developmental Medicine No. 106.* London: Mac Keith Press.

Weaver, L.T. (1988) 'Bowel habit from birth to old age.' *Journal of Pediatric Gastroenterology and Nutrition*, **7**, 637–640.

Whitehead, W.E., Parker, L., Bosmajian, L., Morrill-Corbin, E.D., Middaugh, S., Garwood, M., Cataldo, M.F., Freeman, J. (1986) 'Treatment of fecal incontinence in children with spina bifida: comparison of biofeedback and behavior modification.' *Archives of Physical Medicine and Rehabilitation*, **67**, 218–224.

Yazbeck, S., Schick, E., O'Regan, S. (1987) 'Relevance of constipation to enuresis, urinary tract infection and reflux. A review.' *European Urology*, **13**, 318–321.

11
THE THERAPEUTIC APPROACH TO THE CHILD WITH FEEDING DIFFICULTY: II. MANAGEMENT AND TREATMENT

Lesley Carroll and Sheena Reilly

The feeding process begins when the child is presented with food and liquid and ends with digestion and elimination. It can be divided into five stages: (1) anticipating and preparing to receive food; (2) accepting, orally manipulating and transporting food and/or liquid through the oral cavity; (3) transporting food/liquid into and through the pharynx; (4) transporting food into and through the oesophagus; (5) elimination. Stages 4 and 5 are dealt with in Chapters 10 and 12, while this chapter will concern itself with management of the first three stages. However, it is important to bear in mind that effective management should involve consideration of all five stages

Any therapeutic approach to the child with feeding difficulties must incorporate knowledge of factors other than overt physiological deficits. Understanding the learned cognitive elements of the feeding process is fundamental to the design of any therapeutic intervention. Treatment directed to the physiological mechanisms without regard to the cognitive and behavioural factors is less effective and may create more severe feeding difficulties.

The role of the family, and of the mother in particular, is paramount in the management of feeding difficulties. Although fathers play an equally important role in the development of their children, research has shown that in 90 per cent of families, mothers are solely responsible for this aspect of caretaking (Reilly *et al.* 1993). Providing adequate nutrition for her child is one of the mother's most basic functions. Difficulty in achieving this is perceived as failure and contributes to feelings of inadequacy and depression. In a pilot study of children with cerebral palsy (CP) who had severe feeding problems, approximately 83 per cent of the mothers interviewed had clinically significant psychiatric symptoms (Reilly and Skuse 1992). A more recent community survey predictably revealed a lower, but nonetheless worrying rate. 55 per cent of mothers of preschool children with CP had clinically significant depression (Reilly *et al.* 1993). Even in the school-age child, the mother remains responsible for 75 per cent of the child's nutritional intake (personal data, unpublished) and therefore any intervention programme is likely to be most effective if developed at home with the mother.

Communication between professionals and mothers must be open, balanced and thorough if their mutual skills are to be enhanced and utilized in the children's nutrition. Lack of communication with mothers occurs when feeding is viewed as only a physiological process rather than a complex interrelationship between physiological, environmental, communicative and psychological factors.

117

Children's ability to interact with and control their environment must also be incorporated into treatment programmes and their likes and preferences acknowledged when planning feeding regimes. In advising mothers on adequate nutritional intake other less obvious environmental factors are relevant; for example, involving the child in shopping for food and presenting food attractively are useful in making the child an active partner in meal-times.

Many children with eating and drinking difficulties have physical disabilities that cause marked prolongation of meal-times. Under such circumstances, it is easy for the caretaker to become bored and disinterested and to give negative messages to the child. Thus, many mothers feel they have exhausted all resources and give up at meal-times. Some children with CP have been known to take up to 18 times as long as an unaffected child to eat a single mouthful of food (Gisel and Patrick 1988). The length of the meal-time should be controlled in feeding intervention programmes so that overly long meal-times are avoided whenever possible.

Again, disabled children are often unable to select the food of their choice and/or are not given the opportunity to determine the speed of delivery. Without concentration and awareness from the feeder, the rhythm and anticipatory mechanisms necessary for efficient feeding may be overlooked.

The team
It is clear from the complexity of the physiological processes of feeding that management may involve many different professions (Table 11.1). No one profession is adequately equipped to manage the feeding difficulties of the disabled child single-handedly. Not only is a variety of professionals required; often boundaries merge and each may be dependent on the expertise of the other. The list in Table 11.1 is not exclusive; others such as health visitors, nurses, special needs teachers and care staff often have significant input.

Management strategies
The effective management of any feeding problem depends to a great extent on the accuracy and thoroughness of assessment and investigation. Sometimes, the symptoms observed in children may be misinterpreted. Thus excessive crying, refusing to sit in the chair, and patterns of hyperextension at the commencement of a meal-time may in one child indicate that she is in pain due to gastro-oesophageal reflux, while in another such symptoms may reflect a non-organic cause. For example, they could indicate that she is not hungry, is frightened, prefers to be fed on the carer's lap, or wants pudding instead of a main course.

Communication difficulties
The reasons why communication difficulties can contribute to feeding problems include: early separation; esoteric signals/distorted requests; inability to request food/drink; inability to express preferences; aversion to feeding; and misinterpretation of children's cues.

Separation
The communication difficulties of children with CP can begin in the neonatal period when medical intervention may necessitate separation of the infant from her mother. Infants

TABLE 11.1
**Feeding stages, common problems, and professionals most likely
to be involved in management**

Feeding stages Common problems	Professionals involved
Anticipatory/preparatory	
Communication	Speech and language therapist
Gross motor	Teacher
Appetite	Parents
Nutrition	Occupational therapist
	Physiotherapist
	Psychologist
	Dietitian
	Paediatrician
Oral	
Oral motor dysfunction	Speech and language therapist
Taste/texture	Dentist
Dentition	
Pharyngeal	
Pharyngeal dysfunction	Speech and language therapist
	Radiologist
	Respiratory specialist
Oesophageal	
Gastro-oesophageal reflux	Radiologist
Oesophagitis	Gastroenterologist
	Surgeon
Elimination	
Constipation	Radiologist
Dehydration	Gastroenterologist
	Paediatrician
	Dietitian

undergo their first communication experiences during feeding and respond to events surrounding feeding through movement and behaviour. One of the earliest signals that the normally developing baby gives is a cry indicating hunger. The normal infant's early reflex sound repertoire is quickly translated by the mother into information about her infant's state. When they are separated, the mother is denied opportunities to learn the meaning of the infant's early cries. Equally, the infant will be less familiar with the sight, sound and smell of the mother and will lack the opportunity to learn the effects that her sounds have on her mother's behaviour.

Esoteric signal making
The infant who is physically disabled may be unable to generate early signals of need in the same way as a normal baby. Her cries may be distorted and difficult to interpret. They may fail to become differentiated and related to her needs, such as hunger; this will lead to frustration and confusion for both mother and baby. Under such circumstances, the mother may feel inadequate in responding to her infant.

Inability to request food and drink

Many disabled children have great difficulty with developing speech and hence their non-verbal communication assumes greater importance. In order for this to be effective, awareness of differing facial expression, eye pointing and changes in posture is necessary on the part of the carers.

Aversion to feeding

Hunger, satiety and taste preferences are learned in normal children by the age of 24 months (Harris and Booth 1993). Children who have been nasogastrically or parenterally fed are known to be at risk for developing feeding problems (Geertsma *et al.* 1985). Such children lack the opportunity for learning pleasurable aspects of eating and drinking. Their inability to control and participate in the feeding process gives rise to the behavioural components of feeding difficulty. Food refusal for this or other reasons may be compounded by maternal anxiety. Moreover, food refusal may be used as a protest; the disabled child has fewer ways of expressing displeasure and learns that rejection of food is a powerful tool.

Cues from the child

Some mothers may have difficulty in interpreting and responding to their child's cues; they may be depressed and find the feeding process stressful and unrewarding. In such situations it may be difficult to ensure effective communication during meal-times in order that the child be given choices and time to respond.

Management of communication difficulties

Within the constraints of their disabilities, children should be encouraged to be involved in the preparation of food. Shopping, the smells and sounds of cooking and the anticipation of meal-times are all relevant. In consequence, children may learn to give clearer signals about their needs and wants. This happens initially by a reinforcement of the child's unintentional signals. She may not be able to speak, but can give signals with eye, arm, hand and body movements to indicate her preferences which will eventually be recognized. Thereafter, the child must be offered choices, for example between food and drink (Fig. 11.1). In this way she can learn that she has some control over food and at meal-times.

Meal-times should be as relaxed as possible, with the child included in the family group. She should be given the opportunity to learn a regular routine associated with food and observe that food can be a source of pleasure. Preschool children will imitate their peers and may increase their intake in a group of similar aged children (Birch 1980). Children may also take food and imitate if they see an adult eating.

Children with severe oral, pharyngeal and postural dysfunction are prone to fatigue if meal-times are protracted. This is less likely if meal-times are fixed in length and snacks in between meals are used to ensure adequate caloric intake. Tired children are more likely to protest and become frustrated at meal-times.

Augmentative communication

Some children who are unable to speak benefit from an augmentative method of communica-

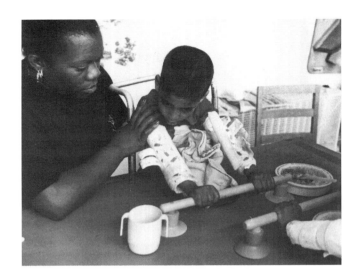

Fig. 11.1. This child indicates his desire for a drink by eye pointing.

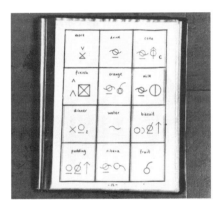

Fig. 11.2. Example of a symbol chart to allow the child to make choices at meal-times.

tion in order to give clear signals. Augmentative systems include signs and symbols (Fig. 11.2) and electronic technology (Fig. 11.3). By using such a system a child can make choices which give her control over the quantity and type of food presented.

Some children can utilize a dedicated speech output device. Augmentative systems are slower than speech and require considerable commitment from parents and carers if they are to be used successfully. However, they can equip the child with a method of positive control enabling her to participate actively in meal-times.

Maternal factors
Facilitating effective communication between mother and child is as important as managing the neurological deficit if feeding difficulties are not to be exacerbated. Parents whose infants are found to be severely disabled have a sense of loss akin to bereavement. Preoccupation

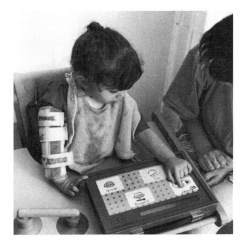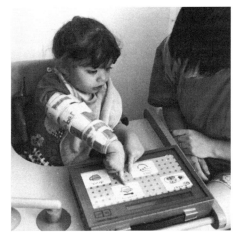

Fig. 11.3. Child using a portable electronic communication aid to choose first her dinner, then pudding.

with their grief may affect their ability to recognize or adapt to their infant's signals. Depression can affect a mother's ability to communicate with and feed her child satisfactorily (Reilly and Skuse 1992). Consideration should be given to meeting the psychological needs of the mother through support, counselling and treatment of depression. The provision of respite care or enlisting support from the extended family so that mothers may be relieved from some meal-times is advantageous.

Teaching the mother to interpret her child's non-verbal cues for food preferences, hunger and satiety can have immediate benefits and lead to more successful communication.

Impairment of motor function

The gross and fine motor dysfunction present in many children with CP and other disabilities contribute to the presence and severity of their feeding problems. The causes are multifactorial and include inadequate postural control, involuntary movements, immobility, an inability to self-feed, and seating difficulties. For functional and safe feeding a stable posture is essential. Children who are unstable feel unsafe and insecure; this can lead to fear and anxiety and may exacerbate difficult behaviour at meal-times.

The position of the head and neck while eating and drinking is critical. For some children with limited oral-motor function, abnormal head posture may predispose to aspiration because of the close interdependency between cranio-cervical posture and pharyngeal airway stability (Bosma 1992). Neck position influences the calibre of the airway; tilting the child's head forward narrows the airway but widens the vallecula space due to the tongue falling forward. In addition, the epiglottis falls backward and is slightly more prominent and overhangs the top of the airway. Whilst the epiglottis in this position can act as a protective mechanism for the airway by diverting food/liquid away from the top of the airway, the vallecula space being enlarged increases the risk of residue accumulating and possible aspiration. In the past this position, termed the 'chin-tuck', has been recommended by therapists for many children but it may not always be appropriate for some children with CP.

Historically, tilting the head backwards has always been discouraged as a posture for children with CP (Meuller 1972). It does have the advantage of facilitating movement of food by gravity, which in some children with poor oral control can be beneficial. Nevertheless, it should be used with caution as it can promote premature overspill into the pharynx prior to triggering the swallow reflex thus increasing the risk of aspiration. As with adults, it is possible to teach children with appropriate cognitive function a supraglottic swallow (Logemann 1986) which enables them to close the airway voluntarily before extending the head. In some cases a combination of head-back posture to facilitate the oral stage followed by chin-tuck can be useful. This is dependent on the child's level of comprehension.

Very occasionally some children are best positioned in a semi-lying position to facilitate the oral and pharyngeal stage. Such a position can prevent aspiration after the swallow which usually occurs because of gravity. If this position is to be used then it is vital to ascertain beforehand that the swallow is safe and to ensure that the child does not have a problem with accumulating residue. The position adopted for meal-times should also take into account the child's communication needs and the comfort of the feeder.

When providing or advising on suitable postures and specialist seating provision it is important to ensure that: (1) the child is stable and positioned with adequate trunk, head, neck and limb support; (2) the position adopted facilitates communication; (3) the environment and position adopted are suitable for developing adaptive feeding skills; (4) the position adopted does not compromise the airway; and (5) the carer is involved in the choice of seat and approves of it.

There is no ideal position that meets the needs of all children with motor disorders. While some benefit greatly from an adaptive seating device, others can be adequately seated and supported on their mother's lap (Fig. 11.4a) especially when they are small, although lap feeding for some children may be disadvantageous by encouraging dependence.

The positions used for eating and drinking should not be restricted to sitting. Some children feed well standing as long as they receive adequate support (Fig. 11.4b). It is not uncommon to find that despite the fact that families have been provided with expensive seating equipment it is not used and is stored away (Reilly and Skuse 1992). Similarly, many carers do not fully understand how the seating should be used; many chairs are complicated with lots of moveable parts and require considerable skill and practice in order to assemble them. In addition, the seating devices should meet the needs of the family and be suitable for their home. Some children require more than one device or seat as the ideal position for playing and learning may be different to that required for feeding. Any seat provided should also meet the needs of the feeder in terms of comfort. A floor seat which suits the child is of no use to the mother if she must lie on the floor in order to feed the child, and nor is one which involves adopting an unnatural and uncomfortable position. Such seats may also encourage abnormal and undesirable head positioning because of the angle at which the spoon is presented.

It is important that the seat provided or position recommended for feeding enables the child to participate in the social aspects of meal-times. In many instances the disabled child

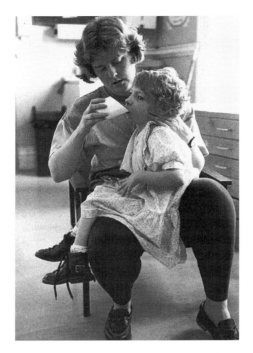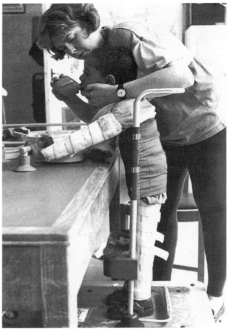

Fig. 11.4. Some disabled children may be fed seated in a carer's lap *(left)*, while others can be fed standing up so long as they are adequately supported *(right)*.

is fed in isolation and does not participate in family meal-time routines. In a study by Reilly *et al.* (1993) 58 per cent of preschool children with CP observed during meal-times at home were fed on their own. In some cases they were fed in another room while their siblings ate elsewhere. Mothers rarely ate with their children. Only 22 per cent of the children seen had regular meal-times with their families or with siblings, although the remaining 20 per cent sometimes had meal-times with friends.

Management of oral and pharyngeal dysfunction

Children with neurological disabilities can have oral, pharyngeal, or oesophageal problems which result in dysphagia. While some may have deficits in just one area, others have dysfunction at more than one level resulting in more complex dysphagia. For example, the consequences of oral dysphagia can produce pharyngeal dysfunction with an inability to form a bolus in the oral cavity leading to premature overspill into the pharynx and predisposition to aspiration. Application of the correct management strategies depends on accurate diagnosis of the underlying deficit.

For ease of discussion, oral and pharyngeal dysfunction will be discussed separately. In practice they should never be considered as independent from each other as both stages in the feeding process are intricately linked.

Oral dysfunction

There are three aspects to the oral dysfunction observed in many children with CP: oral-motor dysfunction, oral sensory dysfunction, and oral structural abnormality. Most clinicians working with disabled children with feeding difficulties are familiar with oral-motor dysfunction but often little attention is paid to the sensory or structural aspects.

ORAL-MOTOR DYSFUNCTION

Eight out of ten preschool children assessed by Reilly *et al.* (1993) had some degree of oral-motor dysfunction. Similarly, Thomas *et al.* (1989) examined 100 young adults with CP and found that 56 per cent had major feeding impairments and a further 13 per cent had minor feeding problems. The children with the most severely affected oral skills are those with spastic or dystonic tetraplegia and associated bulbar involvement.

Traditional descriptions of the difficulties children with CP have with feeding include: excessive tongue thrust, bite reflex (instant bite response on the introduction of anything into the oral cavity), poor lip closure, excessive drooling, and food and liquid loss. However, Reilly *et al.* (1995) and Skuse *et al.* (1995) when attempting to develop a schedule to assess oral-motor skills in infancy could not confirm that these differences occurred consistently or that they were clinically significant. In consequence, they have recommended that oral-motor dysfunction is best described as the serial processes of difficulty accepting food/liquid, in sucking, munching and chewing, and in preparing for and initiating the oral stage of swallowing.

The major reasons why these difficulties occur include: poor bolus formation; poor oral manipulation; limited tongue movements (which may be restricted to immature sucking or squashing movements); limited or no jaw stabilization; inability to create negative pressure inside the oral cavity to collect up food/liquid; inability to close the jaw/lips; no lateral tongue movements; and no rotatory or lateral jaw movements.

The symptoms observed and difficulties the child experiences are dependent to a large degree on the texture of the food/liquid (Stolovitz and Gisel 1991, Reilly and Skuse 1992, Skuse *et al.* 1995). While some children have major oral-motor dysfunction which is evident with all textures (ranging from liquids through purées and solids), others may have difficulties only with one particular texture. In order to manage the resulting difficulties effectively, any evaluation of oral-motor function must therefore incorporate a range of textures. Table 11.2 outlines the common difficulties many children with CP have with different textures and the management strategies that might be adopted.

ORAL SENSORY DYSFUNCTION

Little is known about sensory deficits in children with CP. However, without finely tuned sensory feedback, it would be impossible to bite or chew without constantly biting the tongue, lips or gums (Thexton 1976). The sensory feedback provided by the stimulation of food inside the oral cavity triggers coordinated chewing.

Some children with CP are likely to suffer from oral sensory deficits because of oral deprivation. During critical stages of hand to mouth development they are unable to experience the mouthing activities that normal infants undergo. Subsequently, they can be resistant to oral play, tooth cleaning and so on.

TABLE 11.2
Common oral-motor difficulties experienced by children with cerebral palsy, and possible management strategies

Texture	Type of difficulty	Management strategies
Liquids or thin purées	Food spreads around the mouth	Thicken with a proprietary thickener
	Food pools under the tongue	Change method of delivery (*e.g.* use utensils to adjust flow)
	Incomplete collection (negative pressure)	Adjust flow and pace delivery to match child
	Premature overspill (posterior drooling)	Thermal stimulation (ice chips can be added to increase awareness/sensation)
	Lack of/incomplete jaw stabilization	External support may be given
	Lack of/incomplete lip closure	Stabilize the jaw with fingers
	Excessive liquid loss (anterior drooling)	Varying utensils used can help; support may be given to aid lip closure
Semi-solids (discrete soft lumps)	Food spreads around the mouth	Placement of food directly onto molars or lateral margins of tongue
	Lumps with skins (*e.g.* peas/beans may be particularly difficult)	Avoid
	Food is not chewed but lumps swallowed whole	Consider placement of food
	Food squashed against alveolar ridge	As above/consider discrete lumps or crunchy snack foods that melt with saliva yet provide extra sensation
	Gagging and choking	Offer thicker textures without lumps
Solids (defined hard lumps)	No lateral jaw or tongue movements	Consider placing food directly onto molars or avoiding lumps
	Lumps are spat out	Avoid
	Lumps are swallowed whole	Avoid
	Lumps remain stationary on tongue	Avoid
	Lumps are manipulated but not masticated	Practise without swallowing (*e.g.* dried bananas)

Similarly, prolonged periods of nasogastric feeding may adversely affect the development of oral skills. In such cases children when fed orally have little idea how to manipulate or prepare food for swallowing. Developing a sensitivity to oral stimulation of any sort and a resistance to oral feeding is not uncommon under such circumstances. In order to promote oral sensory function and to avoid oral aversive behaviour, oral stimulation can be provided in the form of mouthing games and employing a range of tastes and textures in the form of toys and mouth swabs and during tooth brushing.

ORAL STRUCTURAL ABNORMALITIES
Studies of children with spasticity have shown an increased incidence of malocclusions (Sandler *et al.* 1974). More recently, Pelegano *et al.* (1994) ascertained that contractures of the temporo-mandibular joint were more common in children with spastic quadriplegia.

The children they studied had increased overjet, decreased overbite and restrictions in mandibular movement. The severity of these abnormalities (especially overbite) correlated with the degree of oral-motor dysfunction, such as loss of food and liquid, coughing and choking, respiratory infections, snoring and snorting and adverse meal-time behaviour. They suggest that new approaches such as orthodontic bracing, mandibular range of motion therapies or surgery may be useful interventions to consider in treating the oral-motor dysfunction seen in many children with CP. Alternative approaches including orthodontic and intra-oral devices have been suggested by others (Haberfellner and Rossiwall 1976, Selley and Boxall 1986).

It is also relevant to consider the height and shape of the hard palate. While many children are able to modify their feeding patterns to compensate for a high arched palate, for others this can cause great difficulty because configuration of the oral cavity is changed and some infants find it more difficult to suck. Also, when solids are introduced food can more easily become lodged in the hard palate. It might be necessary to use special teats for such children and to ensure that no food remains lodged in the hard palate after a meal.

Dental health and hygiene are also important and are often overlooked in management. Many children resist dental care because they dislike any oral stimulation, and the pain from dental caries can contribute to feeding difficulties. Parents need to understand the importance of dental hygiene for disabled children. Each child with CP should have regular access to a paediatric dentist skilled in dealing with neurological problems. Some children require a programme to decrease their sensitivity before this can be carried out.

Pharyngeal dysfunction
Disorders of the pharyngeal stage of swallowing can be diagnosed by clinical examination. Symptoms such as gagging, coughing and choking are often signs that children are experiencing pharyngeal incoordination. Some children, however, show no outward signs of difficulty yet are shown to aspirate (Griggs *et al.* 1989). The gold standard technique for diagnosing such difficulties is the modified barium swallow or videofluoroscopic examination which can also confirm which management strategies are useful in reducing aspiration or laryngeal penetration. It is important to note, however, that some children with suspected recurrent aspiration, on the basis of a history of recurrent chest infections with excessive pharyngeal secretions, do not show evidence of this during videofluoroscopy. Table 11.3 illustrates the common problems and management strategies that can be adopted.

Utensils
Many children with CP can be fed safely with the range of equipment available for unaffected children, but for others some modification or adaptation is needed.

Cups and bottles
There is a wide range of bottles and teats available and there are no hard and fast rules to determine which is the most appropriate. Maternal preference should be encouraged. Bottles which prevent air swallowing are recommended. As many children with CP find sucking difficult, consideration should be given to the early introduction of a cup. Early cups should

TABLE 11.3
Pharyngeal dysfunction: common problems and management strategies

Problem	Management strategy
Delayed swallow reflex	*Thermal stimulation:* use of refrigerated formula and foods. Adding ice chips to drinks. May need to be introduced slowly as some children are hypersensitive to temperature changes *Improve bolus formation in the oral phase:* thicken liquids and purées, pace delivery of bolus, experiment with bolus size
Aspiration before the swallow	*Improve bolus formation in the oral stage* (see above) *Change head position:* chin-tuck may be useful in preventing premature overspill
Aspiration during the swallow	*Increase laryngeal closure and elevation:* chin-tucking, use angle-necked bottle *Create more cohesive bolus:* thicken feeds *Supraglottic swallow*
Aspiration after the swallow	*Dry swallows to clear residue:* if the patient is safe for liquids a small amount of liquid may be given to assist in clearing residue. Note: this should be carefully evaluated before being introduced *Modify food consistency:* feed foods/liquids that cause least amount of residue and/or pooling. Encourage non-nutritive sucking—sometimes encourages dry swallowing and helps to clear residue *Palatal training device:* although some authors report success with these devices, our experience is that their value with severe cases may be limited *Non-oral feeding methods:* may have to be considered if none of the above techniques is successful
Premature pharyngeal overspill	*Modify oral stage:* thicken liquids, change bolus delivery, pace feeds, avoid textures that are problematic
Pharyngeal residue	*Alter head position:* tilting the head back can decrease the size of the vallecular space, reducing the chance of residue building up. However, it should be used with caution
Incoordination between the swallow and ventilatory cycle	*Discourage post-swallow inspiration:* in children with pharyngeal residue a post-swallow inspiration is significant and can lead to aspiration. As far as we are aware no treatment strategy is yet available. In the child who is cognitively aware it is sometimes possible to teach a supraglottic swallow
Nasal regurgitation	*Alter head position:* chin tuck may be useful *Palatal training device* *Surgery*

be soft, smooth and small for maximum comfort to the child. Some babies can manage trainer cups with spouts. These encourage a more mature drinking pattern and ideally should be used as a stage toward using a normal cup. A variety of soft spouted teats are available that can be fitted to either a bottle or a cup and which can therefore smooth the transition from one to the other.

For children who require jaw control or inhibition of tongue movements, sloping cups are best (see Fig. 11.4), and using these the feeder also has more control of the flow of liquid. Excessive spillage can be reduced by the use of lidded cups which control the flow of liquid, in preference to spouted cups. Drinking through a straw is possible for some children and will provide greater independence at meal-times. For training children with poor lip seal around the straw, polythene tubing of varying bore can be used. Straws with non-return valves are also available.

Spoons

Many spoons of varying shapes, sizes and materials are available. Most children with feeding difficulties will find a flatter-bowled spoon easier to manage. Deep bowls prevent children from attempting to take food from the spoon with their upper lip. Steep angles between bowl and handle are not recommended as they encourage the feeder to scrape the food off the spoon against the child's upper teeth, rather than enabling the child to actively take the food.

Children with sensitive mouths, strong bites or jerky head movements should not be fed with metal spoons which may damage the teeth or gums. Plastic or bone spoons are softer and more comfortable (Carroll 1991). Metal spoons can be coated in layers of polythene to reduce pain and dental damage. The size of the spoon should be determined by the size of the child's mouth. For children with very small mouths, plastic spatulas are useful.

Children with feeding difficulties who are admitted to hospital are likely to respond best to familiar spoons, cups, bowls, etc. The range of equipment available on a paediatric ward is usually limited. The child and mother will feel more secure at meal-times if they are encouraged to continue their usual routine. This should include providing favourite, familiar foods whenever possible.

Self-feeding

Clearly all children should be encouraged to be as independent as possible at meal-times. For some children, the physical effort of maintaining stability and initiating spoon to mouth movements may cause a deterioration in oral-motor control and loss of intake. For others, participation in the physical movements involved in self-feeding improve anticipation and cooperation and reduce hypersensitive reactions. Finger-feeding is an important stage of self-feeding which should not be overlooked. A number of aids to self-feeding are available. These include devices which reduce the physical demand needed to raise spoon to mouth and provide independent spoon feeding, and robotic aids which enable switch-users to feed themselves; in both cases considerable oral control is required.

Decision making

It is crucial to decide whether the child with neurological impairment can swallow safely. This issue is addressed in Chapters 8 and 12. Wolff and Glass (1992) have discussed the treatment options for children who aspirate: they propose four approaches.

(1) *Eliminate oral feeding*. This option would be applicable to those children with severe aspiration (on all textures), frequent chest infections and lung damage. For many such children non-oral feeding may be the only treatment option. It is important, however, to emphasize the necessity to maintain oral skills and minimize the development of oral tactile aversions.

(2) *Therapeutic swallowing trials.* For those children who are expected to show improvement and are being maintained on non-oral feeding regimes, therapeutic swallowing trials may be beneficial. Sterile water, rather than food and liquid, should be used to minimize lung damage if aspiration does occur. The aim is to maintain and/or improve swallowing control. It is emphasized that this approach should only be undertaken cautiously and with close medical supervision.

(3) *Small therapeutic feeds.* Some children have less severe aspiration (for example, only with liquids) and reasonable pulmonary status. In such cases the therapeutic aim is to improve and maintain oral and pharyngeal control. The child will receive a full range of tastes and some textures orally, but continue to receive the bulk of her nutrition by tube.

(4) *Full oral feeding using therapeutic techniques.* Occasionally, some children show evidence of trace aspiration or the potential to aspirate, in the absence of any other significant medical problems (no history of chest infections and good lung function). A decision might be made to continue with full oral feeds if therapeutic techniques have demonstrated improvement, *e.g.* if the child has shown considerable improvement with sucking and swallowing liquids and thin purées when thickeners are added. In such cases progress should be monitored carefully and continue under close medical supervision.

REFERENCES

Birch, L.L. (1980) 'Effects of peer models' food choices and eating behaviors on preschoolers' food preferences.' *Child Development*, **51**, 489–496.

Bosma, J. (1992) 'Pharyngeal swallow: basic mechanisms, development and impairments.' *Advances in Otolaryngology—Head and Neck Surgery*, **6**, 225–275.

Carroll, L. (1991) *Mealtimes for Children with Cerebral Palsy.* London: Friends of the Cheyne Centre.

Geertsma, M.A., Hyams, J.S., Pelletier, J.M., Reiter, S. (1985) 'Feeding resistance after parenteral hyperalimentation.' *American Journal of Diseases of Children*, **139**, 255–256.

Gisel, E.G., Patrick, J. (1988) 'Identification of children with cerebral palsy unable to maintain a normal nutritional state.' *Lancet*, **1**, 283–286.

Griggs, C.A., Jones, P.M., Lee, R.E. (1989) 'Videofluoroscopic investigation of feeding disorders of children with multiple handicap.' *Developmental Medicine and Child Neurology*, **31**, 303–308.

Haberfellner, H,. Rossiwall, B. (1976) 'Appliances for treatment of oral sensori-motor disorders.' *American Journal of Physical Medicine*, **56**, 241–248.

Harris, G., Booth, D.A. (1993) 'The nature and management of eating problems in pre-school children.' *In:* Cooper, P., Stein, A. (Eds.) *The Nature and Management of Feeding Problems and Eating Disorders in Young People. Monographs in Clinical Pediatrics.* New York: Harwood Academic, pp. 61–84.

Logemann, J. (1986) *Manual for the Videofluoroscopic Study of Swallowing.* London: Taylor & Francis.

Meuller , H.A. (1972) 'Facilitating feeding and prespeech.' *In:* Pearson, P.H., Williams, C.E. (Eds.) *Physical Therapy Services in the Developmental Disabilities.* Springfield, IL: Charles C. Thomas, pp. 177–191.

Pelegano, J.P., Nowysz, S., Goepferd, S. (1994) 'Temporomandibular joint contracture in spastic quadriplegia: effect on oral-motor skills.' *Developmental Medicine and Child Neurology*, **36**, 487–494.

Reilly, S., Skuse, D. (1992) 'Characteristics and management of feeding problems of young children with cerebral palsy.' *Developmental Medicine and Child Neurology*, **34**, 379–388.

—— —— Poblete, X. (1993) 'The prevalence, aetiology and management of feeding problems in pre-school children with cerebral palsy.' *Report to the Spastics Society, December 1993.*

—— —— Mathisen, B., Wolke, D. (1995) 'The objective rating of oral motor functions during feeding.' *Dysphagia*, **10**, 177–191.

Sandler, E.S., Roberts, M.W., Wojcicki, A.M. (1974) 'Oral manifestations in a group of mentally retarded patients.' *Journal of Dentistry for Children*, **41**, 207–211.

Selley, W.G., Boxall, J. (1986) 'A new way to treat sucking and swallowing difficulties in babies.' *Lancet*, **1**, 1182–1184.

Skuse, D., Stevenson, J., Reilly, S., Mathisen, B. (1995) 'Schedule for oral motor assessment (SOMA): methods of validation.' *Dysphagia*, **10**, 192–202.

Stolovitz, P., Gisel, E.G. (1991) 'Circumoral movements in response to three different food textures in children 6 months to 2 years of age.' *Dysphagia*, **6**, 17–25.

Thexton, A.J. (1976) 'To what extent is mastication programmed and independent of peripheral feedback?' *In:* Anderson, D.J., Mathews, B. (Eds.) *Mastication: Proceedings of a Symposium on the Clinical and Physiological Aspects of Mastication.* Bristol: University of Bristol, pp. 213–220.

Thomas, A.P., Bax, M.C.O., Smyth, D.P.L. (1989) *The Health and Social Needs of Young Adults with Physical Disabilities. Clinics in Developmental Medicine No. 106.* London: Mac Keith Press.

Wolff, L.S., Glass, R.P. (1992) *Feeding and Swallowing Disorders in Infancy: Assessment and Management.* Tucson, AZ: Therapy Skill Builders.

12

THE THERAPEUTIC APPROACH TO THE CHILD WITH FEEDING DIFFICULTY: III. ENTERAL FEEDING

David A. Lloyd and Agostino Pierro

Disabled children with oral-motor dysfunction and feeding difficulties frequently require adjunctive feeding methods. The reasons for this are detailed in Chapters 1 and 3.

This chapter describes adjunctive feeding methods and discusses relevant investigations and their application. Surgical management, including peri- and postoperative complications, are described in detail. Although parenteral nutrition is beyond the remit of this chapter, such intervention very occasionally has a place in the short term nutritional management of disabled children with feeding problems.

Intravenous feeding

In selected patients, intravenous feeding may be a useful adjunct to treatment. If, for instance, gastro-oesophageal reflux (GOR) is severe in a malnourished child, it may be impossible to provide adequate nutrition even with continuous enteral feeding, and supplemental intravenous feeding may be used to make up the deficit. Difficulties in providing enteral access, or profuse and continuous leaking around the gastrostomy tube, may require the use of parenteral nutrition until the stoma has healed or has been reconstructed. As a general rule, intravenous feeding should be used when enteral feeding is likely to be interrupted for more than three days and may be particularly indicated for the restoration of nutritional state prior to major surgery (*e.g.* fundoplication). Nevertheless, enteral feeding is always the preferred method for providing nutrition.

Enteral feeding

Enteral nutrition is defined as the provision of liquid formula diets by tube. The method of feeding neurologically impaired infants and children will vary according to the nature and severity of the disorder. Such children often present with incoordination of chewing and swallowing. If the swallowing abnormality is relatively mild and the airway is safe from risk of aspiration, it is reasonable to begin a programme of oral nutritional rehabilitation. A severe swallowing disorder produces not only an inability to ingest sufficient nutrients, but also a risk of aspirating pharyngeal contents (Sanderson and Walker-Smith 1991). When the patient is consistently unable to take the desired caloric intake orally, adjunctive feeding methods are needed.

Nature and composition of enteral feeds
Enteral feeds can be classified according to their composition: (1) complete polymeric feeds; (2) elemental feeds; or (3) specially formulated feeds. For neurologically impaired infants and children, polymeric diets, which contain whole protein as a nitrogen source, are usually adequate.

To achieve positive nitrogen balance and catch-up growth to an optimal weight, it is often necessary to increase the volume and/or the caloric density of the feeds. In infants, addition of energy supplements is the preferred method of increasing caloric density. This can be achieved by adding extra carbohydrate and fat, usually not exceeding a total of 12 per cent and 5 per cent respectively. In older children, complete proprietary feeds providing 1 kcal/ml may be used (Boyle 1991).

Methods of feeding
Enteral feeds can be given as bolus and/or continuous feeds; the mode of delivery will be determined by the individual patient's needs. Bolus or intermittent feeding has the advantage of stimulating the normal feeding pattern and the secretion of gut hormones. Contraindications to bolus feeding include delayed gastric emptying, vomiting, and respiratory difficulty due to gastric distension (Bentley and Lawson 1988). Enteral feeds can also be given by continuous infusion using enteral feeding pumps. Although these pumps are not as costly or complex as the pumps for intravenous feeding, they need to conform to safety standards (Auty 1988). Constant infusion has the advantage of achieving a higher fluid intake with less risk of gastric distension and aspiration, and improved absorption of nutrients. Nocturnal infusion can be used to supplement daytime feeds, thus causing less inconvenience to parents or nurses. The position of the tube must be checked periodically, and care should be taken to avoid fluid and nutrient overloading. This last point is of critical importance in the care of the disabled child as there is a definite risk of inducing obesity with overenthusiastic enteral feeding (Webb 1980). Obesity must be avoided as it will be an additional burden on the child and on the caretakers, especially if the child is immobile. Supervision by a dietition is important.

Nasogastric tube feeding
Enteral nutrition can be provided via feeding tubes made from polyethylene, polyvinyl chloride, polyurethane or silicone rubber. These tubes enter the gastro-intestinal tract through the nose or can be inserted percutaneously through the abdominal wall. Nasogastric tubes are relatively easily inserted and are usually the method of first choice for enteral feeding. They are used to bypass the oropharynx and deliver the feed directly into the stomach. Before insertion, the tube must be well lubricated. The position of the tip of the tube in the stomach is confirmed by injecting air and auscultating the left upper quadrant of the abdomen. The acidity of the aspirate should be confirmed. The tube is fixed to the cheek by an adhesive tape and is left in place after feeding so as to minimize trauma to the oropharynx. Polyethylene and polyvinyl chloride tubes are stiff and are easier to insert, but need regular replacement every 3–4 days (Moore and Greene 1985). Polyurethane and silicone rubber tubes are softer, more comfortable, remain flexible for weeks and do not need frequent changing.

An introducer may be needed to aid insertion of the tube. To increase the patient's comfort it is advisable to use tubes of the smallest possible external diameter: 5 or 6 French gauge are recommended for infants and 8 French for older children (Moore and Greene 1985).

A nasogastric tube can be used for bolus and/or continuous intragastric feeding. In patients who are unable to take adequate calories by mouth and do not suffer from GOR, the nasogastric tube can be used to supplement oral feeds. These can be given as a bolus after the regular meal in an attempt to promote the sensation of satiety.

In patients with GOR, nutritional rehabilitation can be achieved by a combination of small volume daytime feeds and continuous nasogastric feeds overnight (Ferry *et al.* 1983; Boyle 1989). This can be provided at home. In some cases the reflux resolves following nutritional rehabilitation and oral feeds can be advanced to the desired amount (Boyle 1991).

There are several disadvantages to nasogastric tube feeding. In addition to being un-aesthetic, nasogastric tubes commonly cause discomfort in the nasopharynx, and may block or become displaced distally into the duodenum or proximally into the oesophagus. The presence of the tube may also promote GOR (Flake *et al.* 1991) and chronic bleeding from erosion of the pharyngeal or oesophageal mucosa sufficient to cause an iron deficiency anaemia.

Feeding gastrostomy

The criteria for consideration of insertion of a gastrostomy tube include: (1) Inability to swallow; (2) unsafe swallow or recurrent aspiration; (3) oro-aversive behaviour; (4) prolonged dependence (>6 weeks) on nasogastric tube feeding; (5) prolonged (>40 minutes) oral feed-ing times; or (6) compromised growth. The presence of one or more of these features in a disabled child should lead to a consideration of gastrostomy feeding as the optimal route of enteral nutrition (Boyle 1991, Park *et al.* 1992, Sullivan 1992).

Stamm gastrostomy

The Stamm technique is the established and most widely used method for inserting a tem-porary or long-term gastrostomy tube and can be applied to small infants as well as to older children. It is the operation of choice in patients who have had a previous abdominal opera-tion or who require a fundoplication. It is advisable to use this open technique rather than the percutaneous endoscopic method (see below) if the operator's gastroscopic skills are limited. Although the operation can be performed under sedation and local anaesthesia, general anaesthesia is preferred. The technique consists of a small abdominal incision to expose the body of the stomach. The gastrostomy tube is inserted through an opening made in the anterior wall of the stomach, well proximal to the pylorus to avoid gastric outlet obstruction, and away from the fundus to allow a possible fundoplication in the future. Two concentric purse string sutures are inserted around the gastrostomy tube (Fig. 12.1). The authors pre-fer a Foley catheter, but a de Pezzer or Malecot catheter may also be used. The tube exits through the abdominal wall through a separate stab incision or directly through the laparotomy incision. The stomach is secured to the abdominal wall with non-absorbable sutures around the gastrostomy site to prevent gastric separation from the abdominal wall. The tube is secured

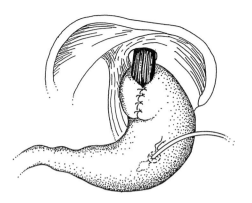

Fig. 12.1. Nissen fundoplication and Stamm gastrostomy.

to the skin at the exit site to prevent displacement. Gastrostomy feeds can usually be started after 24–36 hours.

A gastrostomy tube should not be changed for at least three weeks. If this becomes necessary because of inadvertent removal, a new tube should be inserted promptly taking care to avoid causing gastric separation. It is important to verify the intragastric position of the new tube by contrast X-rays; a small amount of water-soluble contrast is injected through the gastrostomy tube to establish its position and to exclude any leak.

Percutaneous endoscopic gastrostomy (PEG)
In 1980, Gauderer *et al.* described a method for inserting a gastrostomy tube without laparotomy, using a percutaneous technique with endoscopic guidance. With the endoscope *in situ*, the stomach is inflated with air to displace the liver, spleen and colon away from the gastrostomy site. A 16-gauge cannula is introduced through the abdominal wall into the stomach under direct vision via the gastroscope. A guide wire is introduced through the cannula, grasped by the endoscope, and brought out through the mouth (Fig. 12.2*a*). The specially designed gastrostomy tube is attached to the guide wire and pulled through the mouth and oesophagus into the stomach and out through the gastric and abdominal walls (Fig. 12.2*b*). It is held in place by an internal flange and an external bar (Fig. 12.2*c*). The procedure is quick, causes minimal discomfort, does not produce an ileus, and can be performed safely in children with severe musculoskeletal deformities (Gauderer 1991). A relative contraindication to PEG is previous abdominal operations, especially if involving the upper quadrants of the abdomen. There is evidence, however, that a PEG procedure is safe for those children who have a ventriculoperitoneal shunt *in situ* (Graham *et al.* 1993). Enteral feeding can be started 12 hours after insertion of the PEG. The gastrostomy tube may be changed 2–3 months after insertion.

Percutaneous ultrasound-guided gastrostomy
Direct long term access to the stomach can be obtained using a percutaneous non-endoscopic

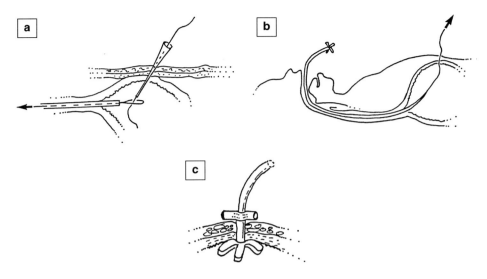

Fig. 12.2. Percutaneous endoscopic gastrostomy (see text for stages).

technique to insert the gastrostomy tube (Cory *et al.* 1988, King *et al.* 1993). Barium or water-soluble contrast is given orally the evening preceding the insertion of the gastrostomy tube to enable the position of the transverse colon in relation to the stomach and the anterior abdominal wall to be determined by fluoroscopy at the time of gastrostomy insertion. Under local anaesthesia, a guide wire is inserted by direct percutaneous transabdominal puncture into the distended stomach, under ultrasound control. An intragastric spiral catheter is inserted over the guidewire.

The advantage of this technique is that general anaesthesia and laparotomy are avoided. The procedure does not allow fixation of the stomach to the anterior abdominal wall, which is of particular importance during the early postoperative healing phase. Experience with this technique is still limited, and the risk of partial gastric separation, leakage and infection is unknown.

Janeway gastrostomy
The Janeway gastrostomy has been advocated for long term tube feeding. This gastrostomy consists of a surgically constructed gastric pedicle tube which is brought out through the abdominal wall as a stoma. The Janeway gastrostomy has the theoretical advantage of being continent, therefore avoiding leakage of gastric content through the stoma and erosion of the surrounding skin. The gastrostomy is suitable for intermittent catheterization thus avoiding the permanent presence of a tube. In practice, stomal continence is difficult to achieve without creating cannulation difficulties. Gastric mucosal prolapse with ischaemia and haemorrhage have been reported (Dudgeon 1993). This technique is rarely used in infants and children.

Gastrostomy button

The gastrostomy button was developed by Gauderer *et al.* (1980) to obviate some of the problems commonly encountered with conventional tubes (see below). The gastrostomy button is made of silicone rubber, is self-retaining and remains flush with the skin. The intragastric portion is similar to a de Pezzer catheter, and a one-way valve prevents reflux of gastric contents. An attached cap closes the device. The button can be inserted 6–8 weeks after a Stamm or percutaneous gastrostomy.

To insert the button, the gastrostomy tube is removed and the thickness of the abdominal wall is measured to enable the appropriately sized button to be selected. This is inserted using an obturator. The procedure may be performed without general anaesthesia, though this may be advisable for young infants. Occasional peristomal complications are reported. Leakage is rare. The button may require changing, usually after 6–9 months, because of valve failure (Dudgeon 1993).

Complications of gastrostomy

Complications may occur after all types of gastrostomy tube insertion and can be life-threatening. The most serious is early separation of the stomach from the anterior abdominal wall, with leakage of gastric contents into the peritoneal cavity. This can result from inadequate fixation of the stomach to the abdominal wall at the time of tube insertion or from early tube replacement. Care must be taken if it becomes necessary to replace the gastrostomy tube within three weeks after insertion, and its position should be confirmed radiologically. Postoperative wound infection and fascial dehiscence can occur after Stamm gastrostomy; this complication is more likely when the tube is brought out through the incision. Complications with the PEG technique are rare, and include gastrocolic fistula and catheter tract infection (Gauderer 1991). Erythema and/or cellulitis after PEG can be avoided by increasing the length of the skin incision to allow easy drainage of any fluid which may accumulate around the gastrostomy (Gauderer 1991) and by avoiding excessive pressure on the skin from the retaining crossbar (Fig. 12.2*c*).

The commonest long term complication of gastrostomy is leakage of gastric content leading to erosion of the skin and discomfort. This may be due to the balloon or flange of the gastrostomy tube slipping into the gastric lumen, allowing seepage of gastric content around the catheter. Gentle traction and impaction of the balloon against the inner side of the stoma may resolve the problem. Pivotal movement of the tube at the exit site, with persistent leakage and skin erosion, can cause a large opening to develop at the stoma site (Gauderer *et al.* 1988). It is advisable to remove the tube for a few days, applying a firm dressing to the stoma to allow it to close partially before reinserting the tube, which must be well secured. Nasogastric tube feeds or intravenous feeding may be required during this period.

Other complications include gastric outlet obstruction due to siting the gastrostomy too near the pylorus or to migration of the tube into the duodenum (Gauderer 1995). The length of the tube protruding from the abdominal wall should be checked periodically to avoid the latter complication. Plastic clips are used to secure the tube and prevent excess movement at the stoma and internal migration of the tube. Less commonly, the catheter balloon may obstruct the oesophagus.

Gastro-oesophageal reflux has been noted following gastrostomy in patients who did not have features of this before the gastrostomy (Jolley *et al*. 1985, Mollitt *et al*. 1985, Langer *et al*. 1988). This is seen particularly in neurologically impaired children. Post-gastrostomy GOR has been also demonstrated in an animal model (Canal *et al*. 1987). Measures recommended to prevent this complication include placing the gastrostomy tube into the lesser curvature (Seekri *et al*. 1991), performing a protective anterior gastropexy (Heij *et al*. 1991), or a prophylactic anti-reflux operation (Jolley *et al*. 1985). We perform an anti-reflux procedure in neurologically impaired children at the time of gastrostomy placement if there is clinical evidence of severe persistent GOR.

Feeding jejunostomy
Delivery of feeds directly into the jejunum is an option for patients with persistent severe GOR who are not suitable for anti-reflux surgery, or in whom an anti-reflux procedure has failed, and in whom continuous intragastric feeding has not been successful. Access to the jejunum can be obtained via the stomach or directly by creation of a tube or open jejunostomy.

Placement of a jejunostomy tube co-axially through a gastrostomy tube was successfully used in 44 patients by Albanese *et al*. (1993) as an alternative to fundoplication. Only four patients had a significant complication (intussusception, 1; continuing GOR, 1; pneumonia, 2). A Roux-en-Y jejunostomy was used by DeCou *et al*. (1993). They closed the end of the jejunal limb around a catheter brought out through the abdominal wall much in the same way as a gastrostomy (6 patients) or by creating a formal jejunostomy (4 patients). The former was found to be more effective for feeding and was associated with fewer complications. A feeding jejunostomy may also be constructed using laparoscopic surgery. This technique takes longer to perform but has the advantages of less pain and more rapid recovery after operation (Eltringham *et al*. 1993).

Gastro-oesophageal reflux
GOR has a multifactorial aetiology and the following variables play a role in its development: incompetence of the anti-reflux barrier provided by the lower oesophageal sphincter; delayed emptying of the stomach; impaired oesophageal clearance; aggressive refluxate; and raised intra-abdominal pressure. Several factors contribute to the high incidence of GOR (15–75 per cent) in neurologically impaired children (Cadman *et al*. 1978, Sondheimer and Morris 1979, Byrne *et al*. 1982). In such children, GOR is probably part of a generalized dysmotility of the foregut, if not the entire intestine (Van Winckel and Robberecht 1993). As a result of neuromuscular incoordination, oesophageal motility and the anti-reflux function of the lower oesophageal sphincter mechanism are impaired. Drugs such as the xanthines, theophylline and caffeine, though having a stimulatory effect on the respiratory system, decrease lower oesophageal sphincter pressure and increase gastric acid secretion (Vandenplas *et al*. 1986). In GOR, gastric emptying may be prolonged. Di Lorenzo *et al*. (1987) found delayed gastric emptying in children over 6 years of age with GOR but not in those under 3 years, while others have reported delayed gastric emptying in 28–50 per cent of patients with GOR, particularly those with neurological impairment (Fonkalsrud *et*

al. 1985, Papaila *et al.* 1989). Moreover, GOR is promoted by nursing children in a supine posture, and by increased intra-abdominal pressure due to seizures or spasticity (Reyes *et al.* 1993).

Complications

OESOPHAGITIS

Several mechanisms exist to protect the oesophageal mucosa from gastric acid. These include effective functioning of the lower oesophageal sphincter pressure, the role of saliva in neutralizing gastric acid and caudad oesophageal peristalsis. Neurologically impaired children who drool excessively can be deprived of the protection afforded by saliva.

Under normal circumstances, oesophageal peristalsis rapidly returns refluxed acid from the lower oesophagus to the stomach. With oesophageal dysmotility, this process is impaired, and there is prolonged exposure of the oesophageal mucosa to gastric acid, leading to peptic oesophagitis. The inflamed oesophageal mucosa may bleed, causing hypochromic anaemia; occasionally bleeding is severe enough to present with acute haematemesis. With chronic inflammation, the oesophageal wall becomes thickened and narrowed and motility is further impaired. In the early stages of the disease the process is reversible, provided the reflux is controlled (Cheu *et al.* 1992). Eventually a permanent fibrous stricture develops, with progressive obstruction of the oesophagus leading to food impaction and regurgitation (Rode *et al.* 1992). Typically, the stricture is short and involves the most distal oesophagus, but occasionally a stricture is found higher in the mid-oesophagus.

Persistent GOR leads to columnar metaplasia of the oesophageal epithelium; this is Barrett's oesophagus. At endoscopy the abnormal mucosa appears as red patches, which on microscopy resemble gastric or intestinal mucosa. In adults, Barrett's oesophagus is associated with a 30- to 40-fold increased risk of oesophageal malignancy, and the prevalence of carcinoma in patients with Barrett's oesophagus is 5–10 per cent (Cheu *et al.* 1992). With the increasing use of oesophageal biopsy in patients with GOR, Barrett's oesophagus is being recognized more frequently in children, but its significance in terms of malignancy is not known. Reports of adenocarcinoma developing in children with Barrett's oesophagus are rare. There is no reliable evidence that effective control of the acid reflux with drugs or fundoplication will allow the Barrett's epithelium to revert to normal (Cheu *et al.* 1992), although this has been reported (Hassall and Weinstein 1992). Continued surveillance of patients with Barrett's oesophagus is essential, by regular oesophagoscopy and biopsy. If dysplasia is identified, the abnormal oesophagus should be resected (Othersen *et al.* 1993).

RESPIRATORY DISEASE

Orenstein and Orenstein (1988) have reviewed the spectrum of respiratory abnormalities associated with GOR. These include aspiration and reflux-induced reflex laryngospasm, reflex bronchospasm and reflex central apnoea. Furthermore, there is an association of GOR with apparently life-threatening events (de Bethmann *et al.* 1993). The respiratory consequences of GOR are covered in detail in Chapter 5.

Neurologically impaired children are often malnourished, especially if feeding is difficult and time-consuming. This is aggravated if there is concurrent GOR (Lewis *et al.* 1994). As a result, the daily intake may be suboptimal, particularly if the child has a raised energy requirement due to hyperactivity or involuntary movements (see Chapter 4).

Clinical features

The diagnosis of GOR is particularly difficult in neurologically impaired children because characteristic clinical features may be absent (Splaingard *et al.* 1988). The cardinal clinical feature of GOR is vomiting during or after feeds. This may be associated with coughing, choking and cyanotic episodes due to aspiration. Acid reflux may cause pain (heartburn), manifesting as restlessness, abnormal movements or refusal to take feeds. Projectile vomiting is not uncommon with GOR, but delayed gastric emptying should be excluded. Other symptoms may reflect the presence of complications, notably oesophagitis (dysphagia, haematemesis), pneumonitis, and apnoea. Sandifer syndrome refers to the strange dystonic twisting movements of the neck which occur in some children during episodes of reflux (Kinsbourne 1964, Sutcliffe 1969). Careful evaluation during feeds given by an experienced carer is needed to distinguish GOR from uncoordinated swallowing as the main cause for the disordered feeding. Since both conditions frequently coexist, a clear distinction is not usually possible on clinical grounds alone.

Refusal to feed (feeding aversion) is a seldom reported consequence of GOR. It is more common in neurologically impaired children and usually is attributed to an inability to swallow. However, among 600 infants with GOR, Dellert *et al.* (1993) identified 25 (4 per cent) in whom resistance to feeding was a prominent feature, either at the time of diagnosis or during treatment. Characteristic features included irritability during feeds with crying, turning the head to avoid the breast or bottle, tongue thrusting to extrude the nipple, and arching. All infants in this study required feeding by tube.

Diagnostic investigations

The various techniques of diagnostic investigation of GOR are listed in Table 12.1. The radiological studies are detailed in Chapter 8.

Clinical management

Table 12.2 indicates a phased therapeutic approach to the management of GOR in children, modified from Vandenplas *et al.* (1993). It is important to emphasize that although the simpler medical modes of management of GOR are often very effective in neurologically normal children, experience has shown them to be very much less effective in neurologically impaired children who will often require surgical intervention.

Traditionally, the mainstay of the management of GOR is to avoid over-distending the stomach by giving more frequent, smaller volume feeds ensuring that daily requirements are met. This approach may be successful in its own right. Frequently, thickening the feeds with gum- or starch-based compounds is advocated. Recent evidence, however, suggests that this may in some circumstances be disadvantageous as the osmotic effects of the thick-

TABLE 12.1
Diagnostic investigations in gastro-oesophageal reflux

Contrast studies	
Advantages:	Direct visualization identifies anatomical defects
Disadvantages:	Insensitive method
Oesophageal pH monitoring	
Advantages:	Current 'gold' standard
	Quantitative assessment
	Indicates contribution of posture and feeding to GOR
Disadvantages:	Requires specialist equipment
	Requires precise positioning of the pH probe
	Prolonged (24 hour) investigation
Oesophagogastroscopy	
Advantages:	Direct inspection of the oesophagus
	Biopsies from the oesophagus and stomach
Disadvantages:	Invasive procedure
	Heavy sedation or general anaesthesia required
Isotope milk scan	
Advantages:	Can help identify aspiration
Disadvantages:	Insensitive technique

ener can cause gastric distension, delayed gastric emptying and therefore exacerbation of reflux. When dietary requirements are not met by frequent small volume feeds, overnight pump-assisted nasogastric tube feeding is sometimes used. However, this may exacerbate reflux and must be used with caution especially in neurologically impaired children (Ferry *et al.* 1983).

For severe GOR and in association with other management methods, continuous feeds by nasogastric tube, gastrostomy or jejunostomy may be required. Intravenous feeding with discontinuation of enteral feeding is necessary for the rare child with particularly severe complications such as recurrent aspiration pneumonia and undernutrition.

POSTURE

The supine horizontal posture increases the risk of GOR. Although Orenstein and Whitington (1983) reported a reduced incidence of GOR in the prone position, this has not been substantiated and a supine semi-recumbent or sitting position is recommended for infants with GOR. This position is easier for oral feeding and allows visual contact with the caretaker and the environment, but does carry a risk of aspiration should severe GOR occur. The posture must be adapted to the needs of the individual child.

ANTACID MEDICATION

Since gastric acid is the cause of the damage to the oesophageal mucosa, it is logical to give antacid therapy. Traditional antacids, such as magnesium trisilicate and aluminium hydroxide, neutralize gastric acid but do not reduce acid production and generally are ineffective. Alginate preparations such as 'Gaviscon' have the additional effect of forming

TABLE 12.2
**A phased therapeutic approach to the treatment and
management of gastro-oesophageal reflux in children**

Phase 1	Position: Supine semi-recumbent or sitting
	Dietary advice
	Thickening agents: Gum-based
	Starch-based
	Antacids (alginic acid)
	Sucralfate
Phase 2	(phase 1 recommendations plus):
	Prokinetic agents: cisapride
	H$_2$-blockers: cimetidine, ranitidine
	Omeprazole
Phase 3	Surgery

a layer on the surface of the gastric contents which theoretically acts as a barrier to reflux and may relieve symptoms in patients with mild oesophagitis. Being thick, alginates may be difficult to give through a tube, which must be flushed through well to prevent occlusion.

Sucralfate, a complex of aluminium hydroxide and sulphated sucrose, protects mucosa from acid–pepsin attack and is an effective treatment for oesophagitis.

The H$_2$-receptor antagonists cimetidine and ranitidine (10–15 mg/kg/day) have been used in patients with GOR especially when oesophageal symptoms predominate (Kelly 1994). One of the drawbacks of the H$_2$-receptor antagonists is the potential for rebound nocturnal acid secretion.

Omeprazole, a proton pump inhibitor, is a more potent inhibitor of acid production and is effective in patients with severe oesophagitis refractory to other antacid therapy (Gunasekaran and Hassall 1993). Experience with omeprazole in children is limited and although it appears to be safe for short term therapy, the long term effects have not been fully determined, particularly the effect of the resultant high circulating gastrin levels.

PROKINETIC DRUGS

Prokinetic drugs increase the tone of the lower oesophageal sphincter and enhance gastric emptying, thereby reducing GOR (McCallum 1990). Metoclopramide improves symptoms in patients with GOR, but a study in infants failed to demonstrate any consistent benefit (Machida *et al*. 1988). Further, metoclopramide has a high incidence of side-effects, including extrapyramidal symptoms. Domperidone, a peripheral dopamine antagonist which acts to increase antroduodenal motility and gastric emptying, has fewer central nervous system side-effects than metoclopramide, but again the effects on the oesophagus and stomach are not consistent (Bines *et al*. 1992).

Cisapride (0.4–1.2 mg/kg/day in three to four doses) is a non-dopamine-receptor blocking, non-cholinergic, prokinetic drug which potentiates acetylcholine in the myenteric plexus; it improves the propulsive motor activity of the oesophagus and small bowel and raises lower oesophageal sphincter pressure, and is effective in patients with severe oesophagitis (Cucchiara *et al.* 1990, Maddern *et al.* 1991). Although about 5 per cent of patients experience transient abdominal cramps, borborygmi or diarrhoea, cisapride does not have the central side-effects of metoclopramide.

Operative management

Operation for GOR should be considered if adequate medical management fails to control symptoms, particularly if there are signs that complications have developed. Although the operative procedures usually used have become standardized, they are nonetheless a major undertaking with potential complications, particularly in a child who has recurrent respiratory infections and postural deformities and is undernourished. Before recommending operation, it is important to confirm that the symptoms are indeed due to GOR and that there has been an adequate trial of medical management. At the same time, operation should not be delayed unnecessarily when medical management clearly is not controlling the GOR, as is commonly the situation with neurologically impaired children. Before operation, a contrast meal and follow through X-ray examination of the proximal gastrointestinal tract should be obtained to exclude an anatomical abnormality such as pyloric stenosis or malrotation, which might be promoting GOR.

NISSEN FUNDOPLICATION

This is the most commonly used operation for GOR in patients of all ages. The essential components of the procedure are approximation of the diaphragmatic crural muscle snugly around the oesophagus, and mobilization of the distal oesophagus to increase the length of the intra-abdominal part, around which the fundus of the stomach is then completely wrapped (see Fig. 12.1). The effects of this are to create an acute angle of His at the oesophago-gastric junction, and to produce a zone of increased pressure around the distal oesophagus. The wrap should be loose, to avoid constricting the oesophagus. A large dilator is therefore placed through the oesophago-gastric junction during the procedure to avoid making the wrap too tight (Donahue *et al.* 1985).

THAL FUNDOPLICATION

The crural muscle is approximated and the oesophagus is mobilized as for the Nissen fundoplication. The anterior wall of the fundus is pulled up in a cranial direction to lie anteriorly over the intra-abdominal oesophagus, to which it is sutured, forming a 180° wrap. This creates an acute angle of His but does not constrict the oesophagus, thus allowing eructation and avoiding the risk of gas bloat. Although a large series with favourable results has been reported by Ashcraft *et al.* (1978), this operation has not been widely used in neurologically impaired patients. An effective modification has been described by Boix-Ochoa (1986).

ANTERIOR GASTROPEXY

This relatively simple procedure, which involves suturing the lesser curve of the stomach to the anterior abdominal wall, is not widely used, although satisfactory results have been reported (Heij *et al.* 1991, Borgstein *et al.* 1994).

Fonkalsrud *et al.* (1989) recommend pyloroplasty for patients with delayed gastric emptying. However, Campbell *et al.* (1989) and Maxson *et al.* (1994) found no advantage from pyloroplasty. There may be a place for pyloroplasty in a few selected patients with objective evidence of delayed gastric emptying and persistent symptoms attributable to this, but there is a risk of precipitating the dumping syndrome (Pittschieler 1991) or at least further complicating an already complex situation (van Kempen *et al.* 1992).

CRICOPHARYNGEAL MYOTOMY

Difficulty in swallowing may occur due to cricopharyngeal dysphagia, which results from spasm or incoordination of the cricopharyngeal muscle. Cricopharyngeal dysphagia may be a primary neurogenic disorder in neurologically impaired children, or may be secondary to GOR. Therefore, careful investigation of the cricopharyngeal muscle is important, including contrast radiology, oesophagoscopy and manometry. GOR must either be excluded, or when present, must be treated. In selected patients with persistent cricopharyngeal spasm, division of the cricopharyngeal muscle may relieve the dysphagia, but in practice this operation is rarely used in children (Henderson 1986).

Complications of fundoplication

OPERATIVE COMPLICATIONS

Fundoplication is a major operation with significant potential complications (Vane *et al.* 1985, Stringel *et al.* 1989, Martinez *et al.* 1992). During the operation the spleen, which lies close to the greater curve of the stomach, may be damaged, leading to bleeding; rarely the spleen may need to be removed (Dedinsky *et al.* 1987). The left hepatic vein is vulnerable to injury during dissection of the oesophagus or during retraction of the left lobe of the liver, leading to acute major bleeding (Smith *et al.* 1992). This is particularly likely if the anatomy is distorted by kyphoscoliosis. Intestinal obstruction due to adhesions has been reported in 3–4.2 per cent of patients following fundoplication, and postoperative intussusception may also occur (Dedinsky *et al.* 1987, Langer *et al.* 1988).

OUTCOME FOLLOWING FUNDOPLICATION

The Nissen fundoplication is the most successful and widely used procedure for controlling GOR, and it relieves symptoms in more than 80 per cent of patients (Rice *et al.* 1991). However, in neurologically impaired patients in particular, this is at a cost of high morbidity and recurrence rates. Postoperative complications have been reported in up to 59 per cent of patients (Dedinsky *et al.* 1987, Spitz *et al.* 1993). Pearl *et al.* (1990) reviewed 234 patients following fundoplication; among the 153 who were neurologically impaired, the incidence of postoperative complications was 26 per cent, compared to 12 per cent for normal children, and the re-operation rate was 19 per cent *vs* 5 per cent for normal children. Reported operative mortality rates for fundoplication range from 0.9 to 3 per cent (Dedinsky *et al.* 1987, Spitz *et al.* 1993), and there is a significant late mortality related to coexisting abnormalities and intra-abdominal complications, notably adhesion obstruction and para-oesophageal hernia (Fonkalsrud *et al.* 1989, Smith *et al.* 1992).

- *Recurrent GOR*. The most frequent complication is recurrence of symptoms due to herniation or failure of the fundoplication wrap (Dedinsky *et al*. 1987). This may occur days or years after the operation. Martinez *et al*. (1992) found that more than 70 per cent of neurologically impaired patients developed symptoms suggestive of recurrent GOR, but in many patients these reflect oesophago-gastric dysfunction. Objective evidence of recurrent reflux following Nissen fundoplication is reported in 6–36 per cent of patients. The incidence of repeat fundoplication ranges from 5 to 15 per cent (Flake *et al*. 1991, Wheatley *et al*. 1991, Martinez *et al*. 1992, Smith *et al*. 1992, Spitz *et al*. 1993). Fundoplication therefore has a significant risk of failure in neurologically impaired children, in addition to which there is a high risk of complications developing.
- *Difficulty in swallowing*. 'Food sticking in the oesophagus' may be due to a pre-existing oesophageal stricture, or may occur as a result of a tight fundoplication. The dysphagia is compounded if there is oesophageal dysmotility (Dedinsky *et al*. 1987) and may be covert in children with severe neurological impairment and pre-existing oral-motor dysfunction. Treatment is dilatation of the distal oesophagus. Even if a stricture is not present, gentle dilatation will stretch the fundoplication and may relieve the dysphagia. The authors prefer balloon dilatation under radiographic control; alternatively, bougies may be used.
- *Gas-bloat syndrome*. This manifests as a feeling of gastric fullness after feeding, and at times is very uncomfortable. It is attributed to inability to burp as a result of the fundoplication, possibly compounded by delayed gastric emptying, so that swallowed air is trapped in the stomach. Reduction of the functional volume of the stomach by the fundoplication wrap may also be a factor. Acute, severe gastric distension can be relieved by passing a nasogastric tube to decompress the stomach, by opening the feeding tube if present or, as Moulis and Vender (1993) reported in a 64-year-old patient, by insertion of a percutaneous endoscopic gastrostomy tube. The problem usually resolves with time. Serious gastric distension leading to gastric rupture has occurred in patients with intestinal obstruction following fundoplication; in this situation, prompt passage of a nasogastric tube is therefore essential.
- *Dumping syndrome*. This infrequent but troublesome complication of fundoplication, which affects normal as well as neurologically impaired children (Rice *et al*. 1991, Veit *et al*. 1994), is due to rapid transit of a hyperosmolar carbohydrate feed from the stomach into the duodenum. The underlying cause is multifactorial. The rate of gastric emptying is increased in some patients after fundoplication (Hinder *et al*. 1989, Pittschieler 1991). Further, the fundic wrap results in a smaller gastric capacity, especially in small infants, and this may promote gastric emptying.

The condition generally improves with time, although this may take several months. It is an extremely frustrating time for parents, and close support by a dietitian as well as the clinician is important. Patients may present with aversion to feeding and require feeding by nasogastric or gastrostomy tube (Di Lorenzo *et al*. 1987). Feeding is followed by retching, abdominal discomfort, irritability, lethargy, pallor, sweating, abdominal distension and watery diarrhoea. The putative aetiology of dumping syndrome is two-fold. First, the hyperosmolar food bolus in the small bowel promotes rapid movement of water into the bowel lumen, resulting in a fall in plasma volume (Ralphs *et al*. 1978). Second, the large carbohydrate load in the duodenum leads to hyperglycaemia; this triggers the insulin response which results in hypoglycaemia.

The diagnosis of dumping syndrome may be confirmed by the glucose tolerance test (GTT). Following a glucose load of 2 g/kg delivered by gastric tube, serial blood sugar measurements over the next two hours will demonstrate the abnormal hyperglycaemic/hypoglycaemic response. A gastric emptying study using a standard feed labelled with ^{99m}Tc sulphur colloid will demonstrate the rapid gastric emptying (Lavine *et al.* 1988). Dumping may be intermittent, and patients with typical symptoms of dumping may have a normal GTT and gastric emptying. In these the diagnosis is presumptive and the tests should be repeated if the response to treatment is not satisfactory.

The symptoms of dumping syndrome may be controlled by altering the method of feeding and adjusting the diet (Caulfield *et al.* 1987). Large bolus feeds should be avoided. Small volume feeds given frequently may be tolerated, but are time consuming to give. Alternatively, small bolus feeds may be given at normal times during the day, supplemented with continuous tube feeds overnight. For patients with severe symptoms, continuous tube feeds may be required with complete avoidance of bolus feeds.

The rate of gastric emptying may be slowed by adding fat to the diet. Different preparations are available, such as Calogen®, an arachis oil based fat emulsion. Long chain fatty acids are more effective than medium chain triglycerides. In addition, slower absorption of glucose may be achieved by providing some of the carbohydrate in a complex form. Khoshoo and co-workers reported two children successfully treated with a combination of safflower oil (Microlipid 50%®) to retard gastric emptying, and uncooked corn starch as a source of carbohydrate (Khoshoo *et al.* 1991, 1994).

• *Retching*. Retching is another infrequently recorded complication following fundoplication and gastrostomy, and is distressing for both patient and parent (Jolley *et al.* 1987, Borowitz and Borowitz 1992). The aetiology is not clear; neurologically impaired children have a widespread disorder of gut motility which may be worsened by fundoplication. Using electrogastrography, Alberto Ravelli (personal communication) has demonstrated that up to 30 per cent of neurologically impaired children have evidence of gastric dysrhythmia (unstable dysrhythmia, bradygastria or tachygastria). Moreover, preliminary data suggest that as many as 83 per cent of neurologically impaired children who have demonstrable preoperative dysrhythmia will go on to develop retching postoperatively. More work needs to be done but electrogastrography may prove to be a useful tool in the preoperative assessment of neurologically impaired children.

Retching may be a manifestation of the dumping syndrome, but can also be due to activation of the emetic reflex in association with delayed gastric emptying and acute gastric distention after bolus feeds. A GTT and gastric emptying study should be done to try to make the distinction.

In the case of gastric retention, the infants typically retch severely but, because of the fundoplication, are unable to vomit and therefore become agitated. Relief may be obtained by decompressing the stomach through the gastrostomy or nasogastric tube, but this is not consistently effective. Giving feeds slowly as small frequent boluses or continuously by tube may avoid gastric distension. Prokinetic agents such as cisapride to stimulate gastric emptying may be useful. Recently we have found Ondansetron (a 5HT$_3$ antagonist) to be effective.

Should an anti-reflux procedure be done at the time of gastrostomy?
During the early 1980s it was common practice for an anti-reflux operation to be done when a feeding gastrostomy tube was inserted (Wesley *et al.* 1981, Jolley *et al.* 1985, Mollitt *et al.* 1985). The rationale for this was the high incidence of GOR in neurologically impaired children (Rice *et al.* 1991), evidence that placement of a Stamm gastrostomy rendered the child prone to GOR (Flake *et al.* 1991), and the assumption that the increased volume of feeds made possible by the gastrostomy would promote latent GOR.

This attitude has changed over the past decade. First, the advent of the PEG procedure made placement of a gastrostomy tube possible without laparotomy. Therefore the anti-reflux operation, which previously had been regarded as an adjunct to gastrostomy formation, became a separate major abdominal operation with significant morbidity. Second, there was evidence from an increasing number of centres that gastrostomy tube placement did not consistently promote GOR, and therefore anti-reflux surgery was not essential in patients who did not have clinical evidence of GOR prior to gastrostomy. In 1988, Langer *et al.* reported that of 50 patients who had gastrostomy alone, 44 per cent developed symptoms of GOR and 34 per cent required fundoplication. Subsequently, fundoplication rates of 14 per cent and 4 per cent in patients who had gastrostomy alone were reported respectively by Wheatley *et al.* (1991) and Flake *et al.* (1991). Preoperative assessment for GOR does not predict which patients will develop GOR after gastrostomy, and some with GOR will improve after gastrostomy alone (Flake *et al.* 1991). Third, there was increasing recognition of the significant morbidity associated with fundoplication. Currently we perform a fundoplication at the time of gastrostomy only if there is clear *clinical* evidence of symptomatic GOR.

REFERENCES

Albanese, C.T., Towbin, R.B., Ulman, I., Lewis, J., Smith, S.D. (1993) 'Percutaneous gastrojejunostomy versus Nissen fundoplication for enteral feeding of the neurologically impaired child with gastroesophageal reflux.' *Journal of Pediatrics*, **123**, 371–375.

Ashcraft, K.W., Goodwin, C.D., Amoury, R.W., McGill, C.W., Holder, T.M. (1978) 'Thal fundoplication: a simple and safe operative treatment for gastroesophageal reflux.' *Journal of Pediatric Surgery*, **13**, 643–647.

Auty, B. (1988) 'Enteral feeding pumps.' *Intensive Therapy and Clinical Monitoring*, **9**, 6–9.

Bentley, D., Lawson, M. (1988) 'Parenteral and enteral nutrition.' *In:* Bentley, D., Lawson, M. (Eds.) *Clinical Nutrition in Paediatric Disorders.* London: Baillière Tindall, pp. 31–41.

Bines, J.E., Quinlan, J-E., Treves, S., Kleinman, R.E., Winter, H.S. (1992) 'Efficacy of domperidone in infants and children with gastroesophageal reflux.' *Journal of Pediatric Gastroenterology and Nutrition*, **14**, 400–405.

Boix-Ochoa, J. (1986) 'Address of honored guest: The physiologic approach to the management of gastric oesophageal reflux.' *Journal of Pediatric Surgery*, **21**, 1032–1039.

Borgstein, E.S., Heij, H.A., Beugelaar, J.D., Ekkelkamp, S., Vos, A. (1994) 'Risks and benefits of antireflux operations in neurologically impaired children.' *European Journal of Pediatrics*, **153**, 248–251.

Borowitz, S.M., Borowitz, K.C. (1992) 'Oral dysfunction following Nissen fundoplication.' *Dysphagia*, **7**, 234–237.

Boyle, J.T. (1989) 'Gastroesophageal reflux in the pediatric patient.' *Gastroenterology Clinics of North America*, **18**, 315–337.

—— (1991) 'Nutritional management of the developmentally disabled child.' *Pediatric Surgery International*, **6**, 76–81.

Byrne, W.J., Euler, A.R., Ashcraft, E., Nash, D.G., Seibert, J.J., Golladay, E.S. (1982) 'Gastroesophageal reflux in the severely retarded who vomit: criteria for and results of surgical intervention in twenty-two patients.' *Surgery*, **91**, 95–98.

147

Cadman, D., Richards, J., Feldman, W. (1978) 'Gastro-esophageal reflux in severely retarded children.' *Developmental Medicine and Child Neurology*, **20**, 95–98.

Campbell, J.R., Gilchrist, B.F., Harrison, M.W. (1989) 'Pyloroplasty in association with Nissen fundoplication in children with neurologic disorders.' *Journal of Pediatric Surgery*, **24**, 375–377.

Canal, D.F., Vane, D.W., Goto, S., Gardner, G.P., Grosfeld, J.L. (1987) 'Reduction of lower esophageal sphincter pressure with Stamm gastrostomy.' *Journal of Pediatric Surgery*, **22**, 54–57.

Caulfield, M.E., Wyllie, R., Firor, H.V., Michener, W. (1987) 'Dumping syndrome in children.' *Journal of Pediatrics*, **110**, 212–215.

Cheu, H.W., Grosfeld, J.L., Heifetz, S.A., Fitzgerald, J., Rescorla, F., West, K. (1992) 'Persistence of Barrett's esophagus in children after antireflux surgery: influence on follow-up care.' *Journal of Pediatric Surgery*, **27**, 260–266.

Cory, D.A., Fitzgerald, J.F., Cohen, M.D. (1988) 'Percutaneous nonendoscopic gastrostomy in children.' *American Journal of Roentgenology*, **151**, 995–997.

Cucchiara, S., Staiano, A., Boccieri, A., De Stefano, M., Capozzi, C., Manzi, G., Camerlingo, F., Paone, F.M. (1990) 'Effects of cisapride on parameters of oesophageal motility and on the prolonged intraoesophageal pH test in infants with gastro-oesophageal reflux disease.' *Gut*, **31**, 21–25.

de Bethmann, O., Couchard, M., de Ajuriaguerra, M., Lucet, V., Cheron, G., Guillon, G., Relier, J.P. (1993) 'Role of gastro-oesophageal reflux and vagal overactivity in apparent life-threatening events: 160 cases.' *Acta Paediatrica*, **82**, Suppl. 389, 102–104.

DeCou, J.M., Shorter, N.A., Karl, S.R. (1993) 'Feeding Roux-en-Y jejunostomy in the management of severely neurologically impaired children.' *Journal of Pediatric Surgery*, **28**, 1276–1279.

Dedinsky, G.K., Vane, D.W., Black, C.T., Turner, M.K., West, K.W., Grosfeld, J.L. (1987) 'Complications and reoperation after Nissen fundoplication in childhood.' *American Journal of Surgery*, **153**, 177–183.

Dellert, S.F., Hyams, J.S., Treem, W.R., Geertsma, M.A. (1993) 'Feeding resistance and gastroesophageal reflux in infancy.' *Journal of Pediatric Gastroenterology and Nutrition*, **17**, 66–71.

Di Lorenzo, C., Piepsz, A., Ham, H., Cadranel, S. (1987) 'Gastric emptying with gastro-oesophageal reflux.' *Archives of Disease in Childhood*, **62**, 449–453.

Donahue, P.E., Samelson, S., Nyhus, L.M., Bombeck, C.T. (1985) 'The floppy Nissen fundoplication. Effective long-term control of pathologic reflux.' *Archives of Surgery*, **120**, 663–668.

Dudgeon, D.L. (1993) 'Lesions of the stomach.' *In:* Ashcraft, K.W., Holder, K.W. (Eds.) *Pediatric Surgery.* Philadelphia: W.B. Saunders, pp. 299–304.

Eltringham, W.K., Roe, A.M., Galloway, S.W., Mountford, R.A., Espiner, H.J. (1993) 'A laparoscopic technique for full thickness intestinal biopsy and feeding jejunostomy.' *Gut*, **34**, 122–124.

Ferry, G.D., Selby, M., Pietro, T.J. (1983) 'Clinical response to short-term nasogastric feeding in infants with gastroesophageal reflux and growth failure.' *Journal of Pediatric Gastroenterology and Nutrition*, **2**, 57–61.

Flake, A.W., Shopene, C., Ziegler, M.M. (1991) 'Anti-reflux gastrointestinal surgery in the neurologically handicapped child.' *Pediatric Surgery International*, **6**, 92–94.

Fonkalsrud, E.W., Ament, M.E., Berquist, W. (1985) 'Surgical management of the gastroesophageal reflux syndrome in childhood.' *Surgery*, **97**, 42–48.

—— Foglia, R.P., Ament, M.E., Berquist, W., Vargas, J. (1989) 'Operative treatment for the gastroesophageal reflux syndrome in children.' *Journal of Pediatric Surgery*, **24**, 525–529.

Gauderer, M.W.L. (1991) 'Percutaneous endoscopic gastrostomy: a 10-year experience with 220 children.' *Journal of Pediatric Surgery*, **26**, 288–292.

—— (1995) 'Gastrostomy.' *In:* Spitz, L., Coran, A.G. (Eds.) *Rob and Smith's Operative Surgery: Pediatric Surgery.* London: Chapman & Hall Medical, pp. 286–297.

—— Ponsky, J.L., Izant, R.J. (1980) 'Gastrostomy without laparotomy: a percutaneous endoscopic technique.' *Journal of Pediatric Surgery*, **15**, 872–875.

—— Olsen, M.M., Stellato, T.A., Dokler, M.L. (1988) 'Feeding gastrostomy button: experience and recommendations.' *Journal of Pediatric Surgery*, **23**, 24–28.

Graham, S.M., Flowers, J.L., Scott, T.R., Lin, F., Rigamonti, D. (1993) 'Safety of percutaneous endoscopic gastrostomy in patients with a ventriculoperitoneal shunt.' *Neurosurgery*, **32**, 932–934.

Gunasekaran, T.S., Hassall, E.G. (1993) 'Efficacy and safety of omeprazole for severe gastroesophageal reflux in children.' *Journal of Pediatrics*, **123**, 148–154.

Hassall, E., Weinstein, W.M. (1992) 'Partial regression of childhood Barrett's esophagus after fundoplication.' *American Journal of Gastroenterology*, **87**, 1506–1512.

148

Heij, H.A., Seldenrijk, C.A., Vos, A. (1991) 'Anterior gastropexy prevents gastrostomy-induced gastroeso-phageal reflux: an experimental study in piglets.' *Journal of Pediatric Surgery*, 26, 557–559.

Henderson, R.D. (1986) 'Gastroesophageal reflux.' *In:* Cummings, C.W., Fredrickson, J.M. (Eds.) *Otolaryngo-logy—Head and Neck Surgery.* St. Louis: C.V. Mosby, pp. 2377–2400.

Hinder, R.A., Stein, H.J., Bremner, C.G., DeMeester, T.R. (1989) 'Relationship of a satisfactory outcome to normalization of delayed gastric emptying after Nissen fundoplication.' *Annals of Surgery*, 210, 458–464.

Jolley, S.G., Smith, E.I., Tunell, W.P. (1985) 'Protective antireflux operation with feeding gastrostomy. Experi-ence with children.' *Annals of Surgery*, 201, 736–740.

—— Tunell, W.P., Leonard, J.C., Hoelzer, D.J., Smith, E.I. (1987) 'Gastric emptying in children with gastro-esophageal reflux. II. The relationship to retching symptoms following antireflux surgery.' *Journal of Pediatric Surgery*, 22, 927–930.

Kelly, D.A. (1994) 'Do H2 receptor antagonists have a therapeutic role in childhood?' *Journal of Pediatric Gastroenterology and Nutrition*, 19, 270–276.

Khoshoo, V., Reifen, R.M., Gold, B.D., Sherman, P.M., Pencharz, P.B. (1991) 'Nutritional manipulation in the management of dumping syndrome.' *Archives of Disease in Childhood*, 66, 1447–1448.

—— Roberts, P.L., Loe, W.A., Golladay, E.S., Pencharz, P.B. (1994) 'Nutritional management of dumping syndrome associated with antireflux surgery.' *Journal of Pediatric Surgery*, 29, 1452–1454.

King, S.J., Chait, P.G., Daneman, A., Pereira, J. (1993) 'Retrograde percutaneous gastrostomy: a prospective study in 57 children.' *Pediatric Radiology*, 23, 23–25.

Kinsbourne, M. (1964) 'Hiatus hernia with contortions of the neck.' *Lancet*, 1, 1058–1059.

Langer, J.C., Wesson, D.E., Ein, S.H., Filler, R.M., Shandling, B., Superina, R.A., Papa, M. (1988) 'Feeding gastrostomy in neurologically impaired children: is an antireflux procedure necessary?' *Journal of Pediatric Gastroenterology and Nutrition*, 7, 837–841.

Lavine, J.E., Hattner, R.S., Heyman, M.B. (1988) 'Dumping in infancy diagnosed by radionuclide gastric emptying technique.' *Journal of Pediatric Gastroenterology and Nutrition*, 7, 614–618.

Lewis, D., Khoshoo, V., Pencharz, P.B., Golladay, E.S. (1994) 'Impact of nutritional rehabilitation on gastro-esophageal reflux in neurologically impaired children.' *Journal of Pediatric Surgery*, 29, 167–170.

Machida, H.M., Forbes, D.A., Gall, D.G., Scott, R.B. (1988) 'Metoclopramide in gastroesophageal reflux of infancy.' *Journal of Pediatrics*, 112, 483–487.

Maddern, G.J., Jamieson, G.G., Myers, J.C., Collins, P.J. (1991) 'Effect of cisapride on delayed gastric emptying in gastro-oesophageal reflux disease.' *Gut*, 32, 470–474.

Martinez, D.A., Ginn-Pease, M.E., Caniano, D.A. (1992) 'Sequelae of antireflux surgery in profoundly dis-abled children.' *Journal of Pediatric Surgery*, 27, 267–71.

Maxson, R.T., Harp, S., Jackson, R.J., Smith, S.D., Wagner, C.W. (1994) 'Delayed gastric emptying in neuro-logically impaired children with gastroesophageal reflux: the role of pyloroplasty.' *Journal of Pediatric Surgery*, 29, 726–729.

McCallum, R.W. (1990) 'Gastric emptying in gastroesophageal reflux and the therapeutic role of prokinetic agents.' *Gastroenterology Clinics of North America*, 19, 551–564.

Mollitt, D.L., Golladay, E.S., Seibert, J.J. (1985) 'Symptomatic gastroesophageal reflux following gastrostomy in neurologically impaired patients.' *Pediatrics*, 75, 1124–1126.

Moore, M.C., Greene, H.L. (1985) 'Tube feeding of infants and children.' *Pediatric Clinics of North America*, 32, 401–417.

Moulis, H., Vender, R.J. (1993) 'Percutaneous endoscopic gastrostomy for treatment of gas-bloat syndrome.' *Gastrointestinal Endoscopy*, 39, 581–583.

Orenstein, S.R., Orenstein, D.M. (1988) 'Gastroesophageal reflux and respiratory disease in children.' *Journal of Pediatrics*, 112, 847–858. [*Erratum in J. Pediatr.,* 113, 578.]

—— Whitington, P.F. (1983) 'Positioning for prevention of infant gastroesophageal reflux.' *Journal of Pedi-atrics*, 103, 534–537.

Othersen, H.B., Ocampo, R.J., Parker, E.F., Smith, C.D., Tagge, E.P. (1993) 'Barrett's esophagus in children. Diagnosis and management.' *Annals of Surgery*, 217, 676–681.

Papaila, J.G., Wilmot, D., Grosfeld, J.L., Rescorla, F.J., West, K.W., Vane, D.W. (1989) 'Increased incidence of delayed gastric emptying in children with gastroesophageal reflux. A prospective evaluation.' *Archives of Surgery*, 124, 933–936.

Park, R.H.R., Allison, M.C., Lang, J., Spence, E., Morris, A.J., Danesh, B.J.Z., Russell, R.I., Mills, P.R. (1992) 'Randomised comparison of percutaneous endoscopic gastrostomy and nasogastric tube feeding in patients with persisting neurological dysphagia.' *British Medical Journal*, 304, 1406–1409.

149

Pearl, R.H., Robie, D.K., Ein, S.H., Shandling, B., Wesson, D.E., Superina, R., Mctaggart, K., Garcia, V.F., O'Connor, J.A., Filler, R.M. (1990) 'Complications of gastroesophageal antireflux surgery in neurologically impaired versus neurologically normal children.' *Journal of Pediatric Surgery*, 25, 1169–1173.

Pittschieler, K. (1991) 'Dumping syndrome after combined pyloroplasty and fundoplication.' *European Journal of Pediatrics*, 150, 410–412.

Ralphs, D.N.L., Thomson, J.P.S., Haynes, S., Lawson-Smith, C., Hobsley, M., Le Quesne, L.P. (1978) 'The relationship between the rate of gastric emptying and the dumping syndrome.' *British Journal of Surgery*, 65, 637–641.

Reyes, A.L., Cash, A.J., Green, S.H., Booth, I.W. (1993) 'Gastrooesophageal reflux in children with cerebral palsy.' *Child: Care, Health and Development*, 19, 109–118.

Rice, H., Seashore, J.H., Touloukian, R.J. (1991) 'Evaluation of Nissen fundoplication in neurologically impaired children.' *Journal of Pediatric Surgery*, 26, 697–701.

Rode, H., Millar, A.J.W., Brown, R.A., Cywes, S. (1992) 'Reflux strictures of the esophagus in children.' *Journal of Pediatric Surgery*, 27, 462–465.

Sanderson, I.R., Walker-Smith, J.A. (1991) 'Enteral feeding.' *In:* McLaren, D.S., Burman, D., Belton, N.R., Williams, A.F. (Eds.) *Textbook of Paediatric Nutrition, 3rd Edn.* Edinburgh: Churchill Livingstone, pp. 321–336.

Seekri, I.K., Rescorla, F.J., Canal, D.F., Zollinger, T.W., Saywell, R., Grosfeld, J.L. (1991) 'Lesser curvature gastrostomy reduces the incidence of postoperative gastroesophageal reflux.' *Journal of Pediatric Surgery*, 26, 982–984.

Smith, C.D., Othersen, H.B., Gogan, N.J., Walker, J.D. (1992) 'Nissen fundoplication in children with profound neurologic disability. High risks and unmet goals.' *Annals of Surgery*, 215, 654–658.

Sondheimer, J.M., Morris, B.A. (1979) 'Gastroesophageal reflux among severely retarded children.' *Journal of Pediatrics*, 94, 710–714.

Spitz, L., Roth, K., Kiely, E.M., Brereton, R.J., Drake, D.P., Milla, P.J. (1993) 'Operation for gastro-oesophageal reflux associated with severe mental retardation.' *Archives of Disease in Childhood*, 68, 347–351.

Splaingard, M.L., Hutchins, B., Sulton, L.D., Chaudhuri, G. (1988) 'Aspiration in rehabilitation patients: videofluoroscopy vs bedside clinical assessment.' *Archives of Physical Medicine and Rehabilitation*, 69, 637–640.

Stringel, G., Delgado, M., Guertin, L., Cook, J.D., Maravilla, A., Worthen, H. (1989) 'Gastrostomy and Nissen fundoplication in neurologically impaired children.' *Journal of Pediatric Surgery*, 24, 1044–1048.

Sullivan, P.B. (1992) 'Gastrostomy and the disabled child.' *Developmental Medicine and Child Neurology*, 34, 552–555.

Sutcliffe, J. (1969) 'Torsion spasms and abnormal postures in children with hiatus hernia: Sandifer's syndrome.' *Progress in Pediatric Radiology*, 2, 190–197.

van Kempen, A.A.M.W., Hoekstra, J.H., Willekens, F.G.J., Kneepkens, C.M.F. (1992) 'Dumping syndrome after combined pyloroplasty and fundoplication.' *European Journal of Pediatrics*, 151, 546. *(Letter.)*

Van Winckel, M., Robberecht, E. (1993) *Journal of Pediatric Surgery*, 28, 279. *(Letter.)*

Vandenplas, Y., De Wolf, D., Sacre, L. (1986) 'Influence of xanthines on gastroesophageal reflux in infants at risk for sudden infant death syndrome.' *Pediatrics*, 77, 807–810.

—— Ashkenazi, A., Belli, D., Boige, N., Bouquet, J., Cadranel, S., Cezard, J.P., Cucchiara, S., Dupont, C., *et al.* (1993) 'A proposition for the diagnosis and treatment of gastro-oesophageal reflux disease in children: a report from a working group on gastro-oesophageal reflux disease.' *European Journal of Pediatrics*, 152, 704–711.

Vane, D.W., Harmel, R.P., King, D.R., Boles, E.T. (1985) 'The effectiveness of Nissen fundoplication in neurologically impaired children with gastroesophageal reflux.' *Surgery*, 98, 662–667.

Veit, F., Heine, R.G., Catto-Smith, A.G. (1994) 'Dumping syndrome after Nissen fundoplication.' *Journal of Paediatrics and Child Health*, 30, 182–185.

Webb, Y. (1980) 'Feeding and nutrition problems of physically and mentally handicapped children in Britain: a report.' *Journal of Human Nutrition*, 34, 281–285.

Wesley, J.R., Coran, A.G., Sarahan, T.M., Klein, M.D., White, S.J. (1981) 'The need for evaluation of gastroesophageal reflux in brain-damaged children referred for feeding gastrostomy.' *Journal of Pediatric Surgery*, 16, 866–871.

Wheatley, M.J., Wesley, J.R., Tkach, D.M., Coran, A.G. (1991) 'Long-term follow-up of brain-damaged children requiring feeding gastrostomy: should an antireflux procedure always be performed?' *Journal of Pediatric Surgery*, 26, 301–304.

150

13
THE ETHICS AND IMPLICATIONS OF TREATMENT PROGRAMMES FOR DISABLED CHILDREN WITH FEEDING DIFFICULTIES

Lewis Rosenbloom and Peter B. Sullivan

Models for the care of children with disabilities include the provision of optimal medical, educational and social help and support following on from comprehensive assessment of their needs. So far as children with feeding difficulties are concerned, this assessment includes an initial evaluation of their nutritional, dietary and feeding requirements, followed by ongoing and periodic reassessment. However, just as with many medical interventions, situations may arise for individual children when the provision of appropriate nutrition has to be set within the context of their overall needs, their prognosis and the perceptions and wishes of their parents and other carers. It is beyond the remit and expertise of the authors to do other than identify the range and complexity of ethical issues that may arise under these circumstances.

Failure of oral feeding in children with severe neurological impairment
The decision to institute nasogastric tube feeding for disabled infants who cannot suck or swallow satisfactorily may initially be taken by nursing staff, for example if a child who has previously been feeding satisfactorily decompensates because of an intercurrent infection. Under such circumstances the principle of feeding by tube may be one that is presented to parents as a necessary and temporary expedient. If thereafter permanent or long term tube feeding is found to be necessary, parents usually perceive that they have no choice but to accede and indeed to acquire the necessary tube feeding skills for themselves. The authors have not hitherto met parents who have elected not to do this, especially if it is demonstrable that oral feeding under such circumstances carries with it a significant risk of aspiration. Their practice therefore has been to accept nasogastric tube feeding as a short or medium term option (preferably for a few weeks at the most), especially if it can be combined with the infant still being fed small amounts, usually of semi-solids, orally without these being aspirated and hence with both child and caretakers retaining some of the pleasure and satisfaction of oral feeding.

The disadvantages of prolonged nasogastric tube feeding, however, have been detailed elsewhere in this volume. If this has become necessary, or looks as though it will become necessary as more than a very temporary expedient in young disabled children, it has become the practice of the authors, at as early a stage as possible, to discuss with parents the requirements for more detailed clinical and investigative assessments and to make clear that a feeding gastrostomy with or without a fundoplication, together with some curtailment of oral feeding, has to be considered and discussed in detail.

The personnel who have introduced these concepts to the parents of patients under the care of the authors include not only paediatricians and paediatric surgeons but also nursing staff, speech and language therapists, dietitians and other parents, and significant potential for confusion and distress has arisen at times. The current practice of the authors therefore is for the implications of the failure to feed orally to be discussed jointly with the parents by a group consisting of paediatrician, speech therapist and dietitian, and thereafter to involve other relevant professionals including the paediatric surgical team.

In taking this approach the reasonableness and appropriateness of proceeding to gastrostomy with or without fundoplication in suitable infants has been accepted. The authors are not aware of specialist children's services in developed countries that take a different view, but nevertheless we do recognize that there is a very wide range of preparedness to be proactive by those services, with the *de facto* implication that many children will be referred late, or sometimes not at all.

It is reasonable to expect that the dissemination of information on the ranges of therapeutic procedures that are available and the publication of audit data will at least produce acceptable practice and referral standards.

A much more difficult situation is that where parents and/or professionals come to the view that the profundity or multiplicity of a child's disabilities are such that gastrostomy or other surgical procedures are unacceptable. The authors believe that there are a very few children for whom this course is appropriate. Indeed, it also applies for other aspects of the care of a small minority of very severely disabled children.

Under such circumstances the authors consult widely with professional colleagues and attempt to reach a consensus with the parents both on the limits of treatment that will be offered to their child and on the details of how this will be effected. For some children this may mean a continuation of oral or nasogastric tube feeding, with the likelihood of aspiration or other complications.

Is it inevitable that very infrequently parents and professionals will disagree on the extent of care to be offered, the most usual scenarios being for parents to request gastrostomy or other treatments which are not thought to be clinically appropriate. One mechanism for attempting to reconcile differences such as these is the use of a children's rights advisory forum or similar grouping.

Such a forum's working method might be based on that of the Human Rights Committee of Pittsburgh Children's Hospital, USA (Michaels and Oliver 1986) and could ensure that independent professional and lay advice on the details, principles and consequences of the management of individual children with very complex and life threatening problems is available for both parents and health care staff.

We recognize nevertheless that from time to time, irreconcilable differences in respect of management will arise which have implications for health care resource utilization and with the potential also for civil and even criminal litigation. The specific issues in the case of Tony Bland (a young man in a persistent vegetative state after receiving injuries in a football crowd accident) that were argued through the English legal system, up to the House of Lords, included ultimate agreement that tube feeding was a component of medical treatment and that a decision to withdraw it was legitimately made in this case by the medical staff who were looking after him. More recently in Britain, the case of Thomas Creedon, a 22-month-old child with severe neurological impairment and said to be blind and deaf has attracted media attention because of the wish of the parents to withhold nutritional support from him (Cranford 1995). It is important to stress that this child is not unconscious and therefore not clinically in a persistent vegetative state, and in the view of the present authors, withholding of artificial feeding from a child like this is unnecessary, inhumane and unethical. Death by dehydration or starvation may be accompanied by considerable and protracted discomfort and pain. To suggest that such treatment represents a potential avenue of management for children with neurological disabilities not in a persistent vegetative state is perilously close to euthanasia and is considered wholly unacceptable by the present authors.

Management of medical and surgical complications of gastrostomy and fundoplication

In general it would appear that the younger the child, or the more neurologically impaired, the greater are the risks of medical and surgical complications of surgical procedures, as detailed in Chapter 12, and it is important that there be a logical and systematic approach to their management.

Thus it is only the minority of the most severely disabled children who require gastrostomy who do not also have clinical and investigative evidence of gastro-oesophageal reflux and a significant risk of aspiration especially when adequate amounts of fluid are introduced into the stomach for the first time after gastrostomy. It follows that a low threshold for considering fundoplication is necessary either at the time of gastrostomy or in the weeks following and that the likelihood that this major surgical procedure will be needed must always be made clear to parents at an early stage. Similarly, those children who are a significant anaesthetic risk because of pre-existing respiratory complications should they have a fundoplication, may not be helped by gastrostomy alone even when performed percutaneously under local anaesthetic because of the increased risk of aspiration that arises once they are given gastrostomy feeds.

The effects on gastrointestinal function following gastrostomy with or without fundoplication are less predictable, and again these are detailed in Chapter 12. Dumping syndrome, malabsorption and gut motility disorders all require to be recognized when they occur and to be treated symptomatically.

Given the inevitable high incidence of complications of what essentially are palliative procedures used in alleviating some of the complications of severe neurological impairment, the authors would make the recommendation that surgically treated children should continue to have available to them a consulting feeding and nutrition team (consisting of, say, a paediatric gastroenterologist, paediatric surgeon and dietitian) whose advice supplements that of the local child neurodisability service. In this way the increasing numbers of children with more severe disabilities who receive gastrostomies can have the benefits and the disadvantages of this still novel approach evaluated over the long term and within the contexts of the whole of their disabilities and the relevant resource implications.

Indications and contra-indications for total parenteral nutrition (TPN)

For both children with neurological impairments and able-bodied children, TPN may be indicated as a short term option when oral or tube feeding cannot be used, and under such circumstances TPN is integral to their overall management.

Difficulties can arise, however, if the decompensation of bowel function fails to remit in the short term. The authors have seen this with some profoundly disabled children who have additional bowel motility or malabsorption problems. Under these circumstances the possible complications of TPN, especially infection and impairment of hepatic function, are more likely to appear and are particularly difficult to manage satisfactorily.

As a consequence of this, the authors have taken the view not normally to offer TPN as what is effectively an end-stage treatment, but rather as something to be considered and offered only if the indications for its use are clearly remediable or reversible.

Problems in older children and adolescents

A significant minority of disabled children, especially those with cerebral palsy, develop increasingly severe feeding difficulties in their second decade. Typically these are individuals who have enjoyed being fed orally but are severely physically disabled, may have some degree of nutritional compromise (although this is rarely severe), have always had some oropharyngeal motor difficulties that skilled parents and other attendants have normally been able to circumvent, and may have been considered to be at risk of aspiration although this has rarely if ever produced symptoms. Then, during later childhood and adolescence, and sometimes associated with an adolescent growth spurt and/or with a worsening kypho-scoliosis, oral feeding becomes slower and more problematic. Food may have to be more finely blended, the duration of feeding times may increase, swallowing may become unpredictable, and aspiration, often unrecognized, can occur. Initially this deterioration may be subtle and insidious and parents and other caretakers perceive it as a behaviour problem or a phase that will pass, so that help may not be sought for some time.

The pattern of service provision in the UK and elsewhere whereby many older disabled children are no longer under regular specialist paediatric supervision as they were when younger, is likely to contribute to this presentation. It is of particular importance therefore that continued multidisciplinary observation of severely disabled children should continue into and through adolescence, with effective handover schemes to adult services being developed and achieved.

Conclusions

This volume has been concerned with two areas, namely nutrition and disability. Throughout, the central role of nutrition—the full meaning of which is expanded through its sister words 'nurture' and 'nourish'—in the care of the disabled child has been emphasized. Too often in the past, nutrition has been neglected or dismissed, with a somewhat fatalistic attitude that it was an irremediable component of the neurological impairment.

While some of the investigations and therapeutic procedures described in this book are likely in time to become dated, the underlying principles will endure. These are simply that nutritional compromise from failure to feed adequately has significant consequences, and is moreover to a degree remediable. Furthermore, when planning remedial approaches it is important to keep in mind the pleasure that both children and their carers receive from oral feeding programmes and to take into account, as far as is possible, the children's own wishes.

It is important that the size and projected increase in the prevalence of the feeding problems of disabled children are appreciated. The upward trend in prevalence of cerebral palsy among low birthweight infants has been noted by a number of workers (Pharoah *et al.* 1987, Hagberg *et al.* 1989, Stanley and Watson 1992). Moreover, it is now recognized that life expectancy of these children may in fact be rather greater than was previously believed. In one study, Hutton *et al.* (1994) found that even severely disabled children had a probability of about 50 per cent of surviving for 27 years or more. Combined with the fact that recent evidence suggests that two-thirds to three-quarters of these individuals will have feeding difficulties, this has considerable implications for the input required to provide for their nutritional needs.

Throughout this volume the authors have advocated a proactive approach to the nutritional needs of the disabled child. Early recognition is crucial, and input is needed from the point at which a child is recognized to have a degree of neurological impairment which is compromising the normal feeding process. Data from the Family Fund data base indicates that disabled children with feeding problems are referred late. In a series of 30, 14 presented over the age of 5 years, nine between the ages of 1 and 5, and only seven before the age of 1 year (M.C.O. Bax, personal communication 1995). Early recognition of likely feeding difficulties must be matched with early intervention with a multidisciplinary team approach to assessment, investigation and therapy.

Principles of management espoused in this volume include detailed assessment of the nature of the feeding difficulties which will help to predict the anticipated future nutritional needs, coupled with dietetic and anthropometric assessment. Such a preliminary assessment will allow decisions to be made about the appropriateness of input from different professionals (speech therapists, dietitians, gastroenterologists) and point the way toward indications for special investigations. Only when such information has been carefully garnered will rational and directed medical and surgical therapy be possible. Clear protocols for the management and investigation of feeding problems in disabled children are needed and will facilitate this process.

A number of questions remain for enquiry, not least of which is the nature of the growth impairment of many disabled children and, in particular, the relative contribution of nutritional and non-nutritional factors. As has been demonstrated elsewhere in this volume, nutritional intervention can effectively improve the ponderal growth of disabled children but has been less successful in influencing linear growth. To what extent as yet unidentified central neurohumoral factors secondary to the underlying brain damage contribute to growth failure remains to be established. More precise measures of gastrointestinal motility are needed for application in this group of children, and more effective drug therapy for disordered gastrointestinal motility. Alternative surgical approaches for the treatment of gastro-oesophageal reflux which have less morbidity than those currently available also need to be developed. In parallel with specific targeted research in these areas, it will be important to evaluate the impact of nutritional interventions in disabled children. This is especially true for the need for evaluation of the impact of a transition to gastrostomy feeding in disabled children.

As far as the ethics of nutritional intervention in children with severe cerebral palsy and other neurological impairments is concerned, it should be noted that such children generally take in enough nutrition to sustain life but not enough to sustain optimum growth and nutritional status. Therefore it is unlikely that nutritional intervention will 'excessively prolong' the life of disabled children. Rather the important principle throughout this volume has been to improve the quality of life of such individuals, and that of their carers.

REFERENCES

Cranford, R.E. (1995) 'Withdrawing artificial feeding from children with brain damage.' *British Medical Journal*, **311**, 464–465.

Hagberg, B., Hagberg, G., Olow, I., von Wendt, L. (1989) 'The changing panorama of cerebral palsy in Sweden. V. The birth year period 1979–82.' *Acta Paediatrica Scandinavica*, **78**, 283–290.

Hutton, J.L., Cooke, T., Pharoah, P.O.D. (1994) 'Life expectancy in children with cerebral palsy.' *British Medical Journal*, **309**, 431–435.

Michaels, R.H., Oliver, T.K. (1986) 'Human Rights consultation: a 12-year experience of a pediatric bioethics committee.' *Pediatrics*, **78**, 566–572.

Pharoah, P.O.D., Cooke, T., Rosenbloom, I., Cooke, R.W.I. (1987) 'Trends in birth prevalence of cerebral palsy.' *Archives of Disease in Childhood*, **62**, 379–384.

Stanley, F.J., Watson, L. (1992) 'Trends in perinatal mortality and cerebral palsy in Western Australia, 1967 to 1985.' *British Medical Journal*, **304**, 1658–1663.

INDEX

A

adolescents, 154
albumin (serum), 65
anaemia, 37, 65–66
antacids
    for gastro-oesophageal reflux, 141–142
    nutrient interactions, 65
anterior gastropexy, 143
anthropometric assessment, 66–72
antibiotics, 65
anticholinergics, 97–98
anticonvulsants, 28
    nutrient interactions, 63, 65
antihistamines, 97, 142
apnoea during feeding, 41, 55
arm length measurement, 68–71
Artane (benzhexol), 97–98
aspiration, 6, 42–43
    assessment, 43–44
    of contrast media, 78–79
    management, 127, 128, 129–130
    pneumonia, 6, 26, 42, 43
aspirin, 65
assessment, 47–61
    aspiration, 43–44
    feeding behaviour, 48–50
    function coordination, 54–57
    gastro-oesophageal reflux, 44, 84–88, 140
    motor behaviour, 50
    nutritional, 62–76
    oral-motor control, 51–52
    swallowing, 53–54
    tactile responses, 50–51
    temperomandibular joint contracture, 52
    tools, 57–59
atropine, 97
autism, 29

B

baclofen, 28
barium swallow, 43–44, 78–83
    gastro-oesophageal reflux assessment, 85–86
behavioural problems, 1, 20, 29
    during feeding, 48–50
benzhexol, 97–98
benzodiazepines, 28
benztropine, 97
Bland, Tony, 152–153
body composition, 72
bone fractures, 35, 63

bottles, 127–128
brain development, 33
    malnutrition and, 33–34
breathing
    during suckling, 15
    see also respiratory consequences
bronchoscopy, 44

C

calcium deficiency, 36, 63, 64–66
caloric requirements, 4, 72–73
cardiovascular consequences, 35–36
causes of feeding problems, 23–32
    behavioural problems, 1, 20, 29, 48–50
    dental problems, 25, 126–127
    drug therapy, 28
    gastrointestinal dysfunction, 26–27
    learning period disruption, 20, 25–26
    neurological problems, 27
    oral-motor dysfunction, 24–25, 51–52, 122–124
    postural deformity, 28
    visual impairment, 29
chewing initiation, 25
cimetidine, 142
cisapride, 142–143
Cogentin (benztropine), 97
communication difficulties, 118–122
communication during feeding, 20
constipation, 27, 106–116
    pureéd food and, 26
    treatment, 112–114
contractures, 52, 126
corticosteroids, 65
coughing during feeding, 41
    assessment, 53
Creedon, Thomas, 153
cricopharyngeal myotomy, 144
cups, 127–129

D

deglutition, *see* swallowing
delayed gastric emptying, 26–27
    investigation, 88–89
dental problems, 25, 126–127
    phenytoin-induced, 28
dentition (normal development), 13
development of eating skills, 11–22
diagnostic imaging, *see* imaging
diazepam, 28
dietitians, 5

docusate, 113
domperidone, 142
drooling, 50–51, 53–54, 92–105
   saliva physiology, 93
   treatment, 95–102
drug therapy, 28
   for constipation, 113–114
   constipation due to, 107
   for drooling, 97–99
   drug–nutrient interactions, 66
   for gastro-oesophageal reflux, 141–143
dumping syndrome, 145–146
duration of meal-times, 2, 23–24, 51, 118
dystonia, 27

E
EDAT (Exeter Dysphagia Assessment Technique),
   58, 84
emotional disorders, 27, 29
energy recommendations, 4, 72–73
enteral feeding, 132–147
   agitation during, 49
   gastrostomy, 4, 6, 134–138, 153
   intravenous feeding as adjunct to, 132
   jejunostomy, 138
   nasogastric tube, 3–4, 133–134
epilepsy, 27
ethical implications, 151–156

F
father of disabled child, 2, 117
fatigue, 28, 49, 120
feeding behaviour
   assessment, 48–50
   skills development, 11–22
feeding refusal, 29, 48, 120
   assessment, 48–49
   in infants, 48
feeding teams/clinics, 47, 118
finger-foods, 129
food refusal, *see* feeding refusal
food types, 19
   pureéd food, 19, 25–26, 29
fundoplication, 143–147

G
gag reflex in infant, 18–19, 25
gas-bloat syndrome, 145
gastrograffin, 79
gastrointestinal dysfunction, 26–27
   investigation, 88–89
   see also gastro-oesophageal reflux
gastro-oesophageal reflux (GOR), 5–6, 26–27, 43,
   138–147
   assessment, 44, 84–85, 140
   barium studies, 85–88

complications, 139–140
   management, 44, 140–147
   pH monitoring, 88, 141
   post-gastrostomy, 138
   recurrent, 145
   scintigraphy, 87–88
   ultrasound studies, 86–87
gastropexy, anterior, 143
gastrostomy, 4, 6, 134–138, 153
   button, 137
   Janeway, 136
   percutaneous, 135–136
   Stamm, 134–135
Gaviscon, 142
glycopyrrolate, 98
growth failure, 2–4, 63
   aggravated by gastro-oesophageal reflux, 140
   anthropometric assessment, 66–72
   oral-motor dysfunction and, 24–25
   see also malnutrition

H
hand control development, 23
head circumference, 67–68
height assessment, 67
Hirschsprung's disease, 108, 112
histamine antagonists, 97, 142
Hugh MacMillan Centre (Toronto), 101
hypoxia, 44

I
imaging, 77–91
   chest CT scan, 43
   EDAT, 58, 84
   gastric emptying, 88–89
   gastro-oesophageal reflux, 84–88
   swallowing, 43–44, 77–84
immune system, 35, 40
innervation of mouth/pharynx, 12
intravenous feeding, 132
iron deficiency, 23, 37, 64–66

J
Janeway gastrostomy, 136
jaw function, 51
jejunostomy, 138
Johns Hopkins Swallowing Center, 77

K
kyphoscoliosis, 40

L
learning difficulties, 27
learning period disruption, 20, 25–26
leg length measurement, 68–71
length measurement, 67

lethargy/sleepiness, 28, 49
life expectancy, 155
lip function, 51–52

M
magnesium deficiency, 41, 64–65
malnutrition, 2–5, 23, 33–39
  constipation and, 27
  nature of, 36–37
  respiratory consequences, 35, 40
management/treatment, 117–131
  constipation, 112–114
  drooling, 95–102
  enteral feeding, 132–150
  ethical implications, 151–156
  gastro-oesophageal reflux, 44, 140–147
metoclopramide, 142
micronutrient deficiency, 36–37, 41, 64–66
  iron, 23, 37, 64–66
mineral deficiency, 36, 41, 63, 64–66
mother of disabled child, 2, 49–50, 117–118
  communication with child, 118–122

N
nasal obstruction in infants, 15
nasogastric feeding, 3–4, 133–134
  oro-aversiveness and, 80, 126
neurological problems, 27
newborn infants
  feeding reflexes, 14
  mouth and pharynx, 12–13
  Nissen fundoplication, 135, 143
NOMAS (Neonatal Oral Motor Assessment Scale), 59
nutritional assessment, 62–76
  anthropometric, 66–72
  deficiency signs, 64
  energy recommendations, 4, 72–73
nutritional consequences, *see* malnutrition

O
obesity risks, 4, 23
  enteral feeding, 133
occupational therapist, 47
oesophageal manometry, 84
oesophagitis (reflux), 26
omeprazole, 142
oral hygiene, 127
oral-motor dysfunction, 24–25, 51–52, 122–124
  assessment, 57–59
  management, 124–127
  see also drooling
oral-motor therapy, 5, 95
oro-aversiveness, 27, 80, 125–126
  assessment, 50–51
osteopenia, 66

P
parents, *see* father; mother
pharyngeal anatomy, 11
phenobarbitone, 65
phenytoin, 28, 65
phosphate deficiency, 41, 65
pneumonia (aspiration), 6, 26, 42, 43
postural deformity, 28
  kyphoscoliosis, 40
pressure sores, 35, 36
preterm infants, 20
  respiratory problems, 40, 41
psychomotor development, 34
pureéd food, 19, 25–26, 29
pyloroplasty, 144

R
ranitidine, 142
reflux, *see* gastro-oesophageal reflux
reflux oesophagitis, 26
refusal to feed, *see* feeding refusal
respiratory consequences, 40–46
  of gastro-oesophageal reflux, 139
  of malnutrition, 35, 40
  see also aspiration
rickets, 63
Robinul (glycopyrrolate), 98
rumination, 26

S
saliva
  physiology, 93
  see also drooling
Sandifer syndrome, 26
scintigraphy studies, 87–89
scopolamine, 97
scurvy, 36
seating devices, 123
self-feeding, 129
sexual abuse, 107
sialorrhoea, *see* drooling
skeletal fractures, 35, 63
skinfold thickness, 71
sleepiness/lethargy, 28, 49, 120
social consequences, 1–2, 49–50
sodium valproate, 28
SOMA (Schedule for Oral-Motor Assessment), 57
speech therapist, 5, 44, 47
spillage of food, 25
spina bifida, 108–109
spoon design, 129
Stamm gastrostomy, 134–135
sucking
  assessment, 54–57
  infant, 14–15
sucralfate, 142

swallowing control, 16–18
  infant, 15
  mature, 15–16
swallowing dysfunction, 41, 52–57, 145
  assessment, 53–54
  imaging, 43–44, 77–84
  management, 127, 128

T
tactile hypersensitivity, 27, 80, 125–126
  assessment, 50–51
teams, 47, 118
teeth, 13
  dental problems, 25, 28, 126–127
texture of food, 52, 125
  pureéd food, 25–26, 29
Thal fundoplication, 143
theophylline, 43
time spent feeding, 2, 23–24, 51, 118
tiredness, 28, 49, 120
tongue
  function, 52
  muscles of, 12

total parenteral nutrition, 154
treatment, see management/treatment
types of food, 19
  pureéd food, 19, 25–26, 29

U
ultrasonography, 82
  gastro-oesophageal reflux studies, 86–87
  swallowing studies, 82–84
utensils, 127–129

V
visual impairment, 29
vitamin deficiency, 36, 64–66
  vitamin D, 63, 64–66

W
weaning, 19
weight assessment, 66–67

X
xanthines, 43
xerostomia, 28